THE PARENT'S GUIDE TO
SPEECH AND
LANGUAGE
PROBLEMS

DEBBIE FEIT
WITH HEIDI M. FELDMAN, M.D., PH.D.

New York   Chicago   San Francisco   Lisbon   London   Madrid   Mexico City
Milan   New Delhi   San Juan   Seoul   Singapore   Sydney   Toronto

The *McGraw·Hill* Companies

Library of Congress Cataloging-in-Publication Data

Feit, Debbie.
    The parent's guide to speech and language problems / Debbie Feit with
Heidi M. Feldman.
            p.   cm.
    Includes index.
    ISBN 978-0-07-148245-5 (alk. paper)
        1. Speech disorders in children—Popular works.   2. Speech therapy for children—
Popular works.   I. Feldman, Heidi M.   II. Title.

RJ496.S7F45   2007
618.92'855—dc22   2007020146

3 4 5 6 7 8 9 10 11 12 13 14 15   DOC/DOC   0 9

ISBN-13: 978-0-07-148245-5
ISBN-10:   0-07-148245-8

This book is printed on acid-free paper.

Contents

Acknowledgments

No parent ever wishes to see her child struggle. Those early months before we had Max's diagnosis—and the challenging ones that followed—are permanently etched in my mind. I can still recall feeling overwhelmed, anxious, and grief-stricken. But never in a million years could I have predicted that I would be able to use this difficult experience to the benefit of others.

Having been a veteran of the therapy waiting room for some years, I quickly became accustomed to coaching other parents through the process of diagnosis and treatment. Whether I was spending time at my kids' preschool, getting my teeth cleaned, or shopping at Target, it seemed everywhere I turned I was running into yet another parent with a concern about his or her child's speech or language development. And being able to help, whether it was with a speech therapist recommendation or an argument to use with an uncooperative insurance company, gave me tremendous satisfaction. To think that this book will reach far more parents looking for answers thrills me beyond belief.

They say it takes a village to raise a child; well, it also takes a village to help that child's mother write a book:

To my children, Max and Ari: Writing this book was one of the hardest things I've ever done. I know it doesn't come close to the amount of work you both put in toward learning to speak. I am inspired by your determination to not let your challenges stand in your way. Thank you for bringing me so much joy—and for letting me interrupt your online Star Wars and Polly Pocket games so I could check my e-mail.

To my husband, Dave Richardson: I could not have gotten through raising two kids with speech disorders, nor writing about them, without you by my side. You have always been a true partner and for that I feel so fortunate. Without your love and support, there would not have been a book. Thank you for helping me realize a dream.

To my parents, Tommye and Sandy Feit: Your undying support, endless faith, and bursting pride—even for a high school math test score of 47—has always given me the confidence to take on new challenges. Your belief in me is the reason for my successes.

To my in-laws, Janet and Alan Richardson: Whether I gave you two weeks' or two minutes' notice, you were ready, willing, and happy to help out with the kids. Without your assistance I might not have been able to complete my work—nor preserve my sanity. Thank you for always being there for me.

To my dear friends, perpetual cheerleaders, and on-call therapists Meredith Browner Lewis, Kim Roth, Michelle Gutman, Lori Harnick (who got me in the game), Conny Coon, Beth Kanter (who made me see the big picture), Barb Sefton, and Mary Jane Michaels: I am so grateful to have you in my life. Thank you, Kim, for the steady supply of barf bags.

To my cousin Rachel Singer: Thank you for getting the ball rolling—and for being there to pick me up after it knocked me flat.

To my sister, Stacy Cohen: Thank you for observing Max's therapy sessions to make sure we were on the right track—and for traveling more than 600 miles in order to do so.

To our speech therapists Jennifer Hill and Diane Nancarrow: I will forever be indebted to you for helping Max and Ari find their voices. And I will always be amazed by the magic you perform on the other side of the observation window.

To Nancy Kaufman: Thank you for looking over the manuscript and for always making time to answer yet another question. I am in awe of the depth of your knowledge and intensity of your passion, and I feel so fortunate to know you. Your center has been—and will always be—a source of comfort for me.

To Dave Uchalik: For showing my son—not to mention his overwhelmed mother—such kindness and patience I will always be appreciative.

To my coauthor, Heidi Feldman: I could not have asked for a better partner on this journey. Thank you, not only for your wisdom, but for your passion as well.

To my agent, Daniel Greenberg: For your persistence, and your faith in me, I will always be thankful.

To my editor, Deborah Brody: You have given me an exceptional gift—the opportunity to help countless parents through a challenging experience. Thank you for making the editing process absolutely painless.

Finally, I am grateful to the many parents, speech therapists, and other professionals who took the time to share their experiences and expertise with me. This book would not have been complete without their contributions.

1

My Child Doesn't Have a Problem . . . Does He? Coming to Terms with Your Concerns

I never thought there was any problem.

Between talking with our pediatrician, reading all the parenting magazines, and studying every book in the *What to Expect* series, I felt confident in understanding what normal childhood development looked like. It seemed my son, Max, knew, too, as he hit every developmental milestone on target. Well, almost every one.

At two and a half years old, Max spoke fewer than ten words: mama, dada, wow, oh no, what's that, hi. His main form of communication was shrieking, hitting, and when those proved unsuccessful, banging his head against the wall. He was prone to severe tantrums, and an otherwise minor infraction such as putting on the wrong video often resulted in an outburst so intense and prolonged it was as if Max was lost, trapped in his own hysteria. Routine activities such as brushing his teeth or giving him a bath were traumatic. And it wasn't uncommon for him to wake up five or six times during the night, often screaming.

I considered a multitude of explanations for his behavior. At one especially low point, my husband came home to find me sobbing in front of the computer; a surf on the Net had left me convinced that Max was autistic.

It was in November of 2001—Max was twenty-eight months old—that he was given an official diagnosis: apraxia. It's a neurological speech disorder that causes motor planning difficulties. This meant that even though Max's brain knew exactly what he wanted to say, it had trouble coordinating Max's lips, jaw, and tongue to work together to produce speech. When other children his age were stringing together two- and three-word phrases, Max struggled to say simple vowel sounds.

Treatment for apraxia is intensive; Max would need four days a week of speech therapy if we were to see significant improvement. And though apraxia may have been Max's official diagnosis, his ability to speak wasn't the only thing being affected: my career, my mental health, and my marriage all suffered. I spent many days in and out of tears, mourning for my child and the bumpy, unknown road that lay ahead of him. Emotional exhaustion, the logistics of getting Max to therapy, and my obsessive focus on him forced me to leave a job I loved. The strain of having a child with special needs wore on my marriage and pulled us apart at a time when, more than ever, we needed to support each other.

But I found comfort as Max's vocabulary got bigger and his sentences grew longer. As his ability to communicate improved, so, too, did his behavioral issues. I knew he would be OK in the end, and seeing his progress made it easier to handle the news two years later when his sister, Ari, received the same diagnosis.

My family is far from alone in living with the challenges of children with communication problems. Max and Ari are just two of the three to six million children in the United States with a speech or language disorder.

Some parents, like myself, didn't have much concern in the beginning.

"A little before Adam was two years old, we started noticing that he understood things, but never repeated or imitated words," says mom Dee. "But we didn't think much of it. We figured he was a second child, and a boy at that, so perhaps he was just a late talker."

"It took someone else being more aware of things for us to realize there was a problem that needed to be dealt with," says mom Mary. "At first we thought everyone was crazy because Karisa seemed normal in so many ways; she was just a bit late."

Others knew in their gut long before a professional delivered a diagnosis.

"I first became concerned about Decker's speech development at around thirteen months," says mom Frith. "He had a cousin who was only a month older and he was already very verbal. I know you aren't supposed to compare kids, but I also had this gut sense that he just wasn't vocalizing the way he was supposed to by that age."

"People thought I was crazy and should just let her *be*," says Rachel of her daughter Maya. "But I knew I had to go on my gut reaction and do something about it."

If you're reading this book, it probably means one of two things. Either you have concerns about your child's speech and language development. Or someone else—your mother, father-in-law, or some other person with a vested interest in your child (and perhaps an opinion of your parenting skills)—does. For me, it was the latter. It wasn't so much Max's lack of words that prompted us to seek an evaluation so much as it was my mother's propensity to use hers.

She'd bring up Max's speech again and again, and each time I thought she was being ridiculous. Max had words; just not that many. I knew that normal language development could occur up until two years of age. I didn't want to be one of those parents who pushed her child to do something he wasn't ready to do. If Max wasn't in a rush, I wouldn't be either.

Admittedly, I had mixed feelings about what my mom said. I was certain there was nothing wrong with Max's speech but . . . what if she was right? For nearly twenty years, she was an administrator of a school for children with developmental delays, so I recognized that she knew what a child with delays looked like. But in my stubborn mind all I heard was a mother's criticism of her daughter's parenting skills.

When questions about Max's speech started coming from my sister, Stacy, I listened more patiently. She was a teacher at our mom's school and part of her job was referring children for speech evaluations. I still wasn't worried that Max wasn't talking, but I feared my mother wouldn't stop. The evaluation, if nothing else, I figured, would get her off my back.

So if you're like me and it was someone else who raised questions about your child's communication, trust me, I understand. And if that was the case, chances are pretty good that you didn't pick up this book so much as it was thrust upon you. Whether you purchased it of your own accord or had it dropped into your lap, the important thing is that you're here. Because the earlier you determine if your child has a speech or language problem, and the earlier you treat it, the greater your child's chances are of overcoming it.

I know it's scary to think your child might have a problem; I've been through the diagnosis dance far more times than I care to remember. I know what it's like to overanalyze every sound (or lack thereof) and movement my child makes, to question his future, and to cry off and on for days on end. I know what it's like to have my life uprooted and my career brought to a halt because of my child's newly discovered special needs. I know what it's like to listen to a friend talk about her sixteen-month-old's extensive vocabulary and feel a sharp pang in my chest. It's anxiety provoking and overwhelming, and it's not fair.

But the important thing is that you're on your way to helping your child and getting her whatever services she may need.

For those with a pediatrician/spouse/friend who insists there's nothing to worry about and that you should just give your child time to develop, the next chapter discusses the importance of early intervention—and listening to your gut. Be sure to make copies for the naysayers in your life. Chapter 3 introduces you to the professionals you may come across as you seek information and treatment, while the next few detail the different diagnoses and their respective therapeutic approaches. You'll learn about choosing the right speech therapist as well as a variety of complementary therapies available. We'll give you a heads up on the different ways your child's diagnosis may impact your life, as well as strategies for coping with the challenge. Overwhelmed by dealing with the bureaucracies of your child's school and insurance company? Chapters 10 and 11 will guide you, step-by-step, through the process of getting your child what he needs. Finally, you'll hear advice from seasoned experts—parents, just like you, who have already traveled down this road.

When I was first plunged into the world of speech and language disorders, I didn't have a book to guide me through the process. What I had was my cousin Rachel. It was Rachel who put me in touch with the speech therapist who gave us Max's apraxia diagnosis. It was Rachel who explained how the early intervention system worked. And it was Rachel who hugged me tight and listened to me cry once all the overwhelming information and emotion finally caught up with me.

I was fortunate to have the advice and support of someone who had already been down this path; but not everyone does, and that is why I decided to write this book. So that all parents could benefit from the experience and guidance of someone who has already been down that road. And while no one turns to a book for a hug, I hope you find in these pages the understanding and support from a parent just like you.

Despite many parts of this book being written in the first person, it has, in fact, two authors. While my goal for this book was to offer parent-to-parent advice, it was just as important to do it accurately and under the guidance of a professional. So while the voice of this book may be Debbie's, it is backed by Heidi's years of experience as a developmental-behavioral pediatrician, child development expert, and language development researcher.

Whether you're just starting your journey or have received a diagnosis and are well down the path, you'll find in these pages the knowledge you seek to help your child and the comfort you need during an often confusing and intense time.

A WORD ON DEVELOPMENTAL CHARTS

They are everywhere. At the doctor's office. In the schools. In just about any book on child development. Flip ahead a page. See? There it is.

The thing is, there can be tremendous comfort found within all those little boxes. Your fourteen-month-old isn't walking yet? No problem. According to the chart, anything up to sixteen months is considered normal development. Your two-month-old won't hold her rattle? Forget about it—she's not expected to for another three boxes.

But there can also be much anxiety, especially when your child's age is in one box and her abilities are three boxes over to the left. Remember, these charts are just guidelines. Hard as it may sometimes be, try to strike a balance between their keeping you informed and making you insane. Yes, it can be discouraging—even devastating—to realize your child isn't reaching a milestone at the same time as her peers. Trust me, I've been there. My son Max spoke fewer than ten words when his peers had between fifty and two hundred. Understanding that he should have had more words was an invaluable clue that something was not right. Even after I'd been immersed in the world of speech therapy for two years and considered myself well-versed in language development, it took yet another chart to make me realize my daughter, Ari, was heading down the same path we were already traveling with Max.

Despite the anxiety they can cause—not to mention the tears they can induce (they did for me)—developmental charts, parenting magazines, and all those comparative conversations with your fellow parents play a key role in keeping on top of your child's development. By knowing when she is expected to achieve a particular goal, you're in the best position to catch a problem and seek the appropriate help in a timely manner.

That said, the range of normal language development is extremely broad, especially at younger ages, and not every child will fit neatly

Language Development Chart

	Receptive Language	Expressive Language	Social Skills
In the first month of life, most newborns will:	Startle in response to loud noises Indicate they detect sound by widening eyes, blinking, changing facial expressions, or moving their body Increase or decrease sucking behavior in response to new sound or change in ongoing sounds Turn his head toward a speaker or sound Stop crying when someone talks to him	Cry to make his needs known	Look at the face of people close by Snuggle into a parent's neck when held upright and against the chest Snuggle into a parent's torso when held horizontal in the parent's arms Track the human face as it moves side to side
From 1 through 3 months, most infants will:	Quiet in response to sounds and voices	Begin to make vowel sounds, also known as cooing Begin to vocalize in response to a speaker Cry, often in the late afternoon or when overstimulated Cry differently for hunger, anger, and other needs	Smile in response to a speaker Track the human face as it moves side to side and up and down

(continued on next page)

Language Development Chart (continued)

	Receptive Language	Expressive Language	Social Skills
From 4 through 5 months, most infants will:	Look directly at a speaker Look for the source of new sounds or speakers Notice toys that make sounds	Coo responsively with another person Chuckle, gurgle, and laugh out loud Vary vocal pitch and intonation Blow raspberries	Smile readily at people in the environment Respond differently to caregivers and strangers
From 6 through 8 months, most infants will:	Show recognition of his own name Recognize words associated with physical gestures (such as saying *hi*) by responding with the appropriate gesture (waving) Turn to look at the appropriate parent in response to *mama* or *dada*	Add consonants to vocalization, also known as babbling Imitate actions and familiar sounds Vocalize readily to another person	Show awareness or anxiety with strangers Attend to music and songs Sit without support and play with toys Engage in give-and-take activities, such as rolling a ball back and forth
From 9 through 11 months, most infants will:	Briefly stop behavior when told *no* Look at a family member when named Turn when called by name	Babble different sounds including *m,n,t,d,b,p,* and *z* Begin to add sentence-like intonation to his babbling, called jargon Point to an interesting object or event Verbalize a social routine, such as say *hi* or *bye* Say *dada* in response to being told *say daddy*	Play pat-a-cake and peek-a-boo Share a joint focus of attention with another person Direct others with pats, pulls, and pushes, maybe even points Expand the number of routines they follow

		Have one or more words such as *bye-bye, mama, dada*	Acknowledge others' speech with eye contact, speech, or by repeating the word that was spoken
From 12 through 14 months, most toddlers will:	Understand that when adults point it directs his attention to an object or person Look at an object or two when they are named Clap and wave reliably on command	Point to a desired object Say *all gone* and ask for *more* Imitate some words Increase use of sentence-like intonation in jargon Use 3–20 single words, especially sound effects (*uh oh*), animal names (*doggie*) and animal sounds (*bow-wow*) Protest by shaking his head or moving away	
From 15 through 18 months, most toddlers will:	Give an object upon request Follow simple commands such as *roll the ball* or *get your shoes* Look at or point to objects when named Understand many words, particularly people, common objects, foods, and drinks	Say more words every month, but lose a couple of words as new ones emerge Use immature forms for some words, such as *baba* for bottle or *wawa* for water Sometimes use words in idiosyncratic ways, such as using *dog* for dogs, cats, horses, cows, and birds Mimic environmental sounds (*meow, vrooom, neigh*) Say no to requests	Smile when successfully completing a task Register when a parent says no and then continue with the forbidden activity anyway
	Respond to *in* and *on* Point to one or two body parts Have a receptive vocabulary far larger than their expressive vocabulary		

(continued on next page)

Language Development Chart (continued)

	Receptive Language	Expressive Language	Social Skills
From 18 through 24 months, most toddlers will:	Point to five body parts Shake or nod their head in response to yes and no questions Understand about 300 words Listen as pictures are named Follow two-step commands (*Get your shoes and bring them to mommy.*)	Say 50 words Name familiar objects Say two-word phrases, such as *mommy sock* to mean *mommy is putting on my sock* Use his own name when referring to himself Produce consonant-vowel-consonant words, such as *cat* and *man* Use commands such as *move*	Engage in pretend play (talking on the phone, feeding a baby)
From 2 through 2.5 years, most toddlers will:	Understand concepts such as *one* and *all* Understand about 500 words Understand concepts such as *big* and *little*	Say 200 words Omit some final consonants Substitute *w* for *r* (*wed* for *red*), *y* for *l* (*lello* for *yellow*) and reduce consonant blends such as *st* to *s* or *t* (*sep* or *tep* for *step*) Begin to ask and answer *what* and *where* questions Use some regular plurals Ask basic questions, but usually through intonation (*Daddy gone?*) rather than with proper grammar (*Where did Daddy go?*) Ask for help when having trouble with a task	Request help with brushing his teeth and toileting Sing familiar songs with an adult

From 2.5 through 3 years, most toddlers will:	Understand about 900 words Point to pictures of common objects described by their use (ask *What keeps our food cold?* and he'll point to a refrigerator)	Say 500 words Know third-person pronouns (he, she, theirs, him, its) Say whether they are a boy or girl Clearly articulate *p,m,n,w,*and *h* Refer to himself by his own name Use pronouns (*me, you, mine*) Make negative statements (*no eat candy* to mean don't eat candy before dinner) Are understood by strangers at least half the time Begin to use possessives such as *mine*	Begin to talk about past experiences and events Describe what he is doing while playing or engaged in an activity (*I building tower. I eating sandwich.*)
From 3 through 3.5 years, most young pre-schoolers will:	Understand about 1,200 words Respond to two unrelated commands (*Put the book on the shelf and go get your shoes.*)	Say 800 words Count by rote to five Name primary colors Use regular past tense forms (*I went to the zoo yesterday.*) Answer simple questions such as *what, who, why,* and *how many?* Begin to ask *why*, often incessantly Use final consonants most of the time	Use complex speech interactions with other kids, such as negotiating roles when playing house

(continued on next page)

Language Development Chart (continued)

	Receptive Language	Expressive Language	Social Skills
From 3.5 through 4 years, most pre-schoolers will:	Understand 1,500–2,000 words Know *in front of* and *behind* Respond to three-step commands	Count five objects Tell own age and full name Usually be understood by people outside the family Do simple verbal analogies (*Daddy is a man, Mommy is a ___*) Clearly articulate *b,d,k,g,f,y* Tell how common objects are used Use contractions	Repeat rhymes and songs Sort objects into categories but may not be able to label them Recognize when information is incorrect and protest verbally (*The sky's not orange, Mommy!*) Organize pretend games
From 4 through 5 years, most pre-schoolers will:	Understand 2,000–2,800 words	Say about 1,500–2,000 words Misarticulate a few difficult blends (*top* for *stop*, *geen* for *green*) Begin to use irregular plurals (*feet* instead of *feets* or *foots*) Play with words and create her own rhyming words Tell familiar stories without picture cues Generate complex sentences (*We went to the store and bought milk. He hurt his knee because he fell off his bike.*) Know *between, above, below, top,* and *bottom* Know *heavy/light* and *loud/soft*	Identify *first, last, middle* Talk about her own feelings Use socially common expressions ("I don't care") Use pictures to "read" a story Understand seasons and what you do in each one Pay attention to a short story and answer simple questions about it Tell stories that stick to a topic Sound clear like other children's voices Seek answers to meaningful questions such as *Why did that happen?*

From 5 through 7 years, most grade schoolers will:	Understand almost all of what they hear, consistent with their understanding of the world Understand more/less, yesterday/tomorrow, most/least	Count 20 objects Name the weekdays in order Tell the month and day of her birthday Tell her street name and town Use irregular plurals consistently (*children, mice, women*) Articulate *t, ing, r, l,* and the voiceless *th, ch, sh,* and *j* Have mastered *f, v, sh, zh, th,* and *l* Use all pronouns consistently Use irregular comparatives (*good, better, best*) Use the passive voice (*My friend Mark was bitten by a dog.*) State similarities and differences between objects	Make few consonant omissions or substitutions Use possessives consistently Be understood by familiar listeners most of the time	Use mild slang and profanity Tell simple jokes Express anger with nonaggressive words instead of physical actions (*That makes me angry.*) Become aware of mistakes in other people's speech Tell connected stories about a picture, seeing relationships between objects and happenings Have completely intelligible and socially useful speech Become interested in learning, productivity, and reading

Note: the information in this chart is based on milestones for which 75 percent to 90 percent of children in each age group are capable.

Parent to Parent

"Most of my friends and family, as well as my pediatrician, downplayed my fears when Hannah was eighteen months old. If it hadn't been for the charts, I might have backed down and doubted my instincts. As it was, I stuck to my guns, chart in hand, and demanded the speech evaluation when she turned two. Good thing, too, because she was diagnosed with apraxia and has benefited greatly from early intervention.

—Melissa, mom to seven-year-old Hannah, apraxia
(Cincinnati, Ohio)

"Any developmental chart is only as good as the professional who interprets the information for you. Children can be below the guidelines and still be in the normal range—or have the potential to be in the normal range.

"No one was certain my son had a problem when he was eighteen months old. But with our pediatrician's advice, we kept an eye on it and started the long process of having him evaluated. Luckily, we didn't waste valuable time getting started. And it all began with a chart."

—Liza, mom to four-and-a-half-year-old Jackson, apraxia, mild dysarthria
(Coatesville, Indiana)

"I've always found the charts pretty depressing. My kids were always soooooo far behind. Still are. I've developed a philosophy that life is a marathon, not a sprint, and that the getting there is more important than the goal. It's still hard, though, to sit in IEP [Individualized Education Program] meetings and see results of tests that show how many milestones are missing. The charts are a necessary evil, I think, but I try not to pay too much attention."

—Terri, adoptive mom to sixteen-year-old Elena, language-based learning
disorders, and thirteen-year-old Andrew, fetal alcohol effects
(Clifton, New Jersey)

"It was stressful to see how 'behind' James was for his age. Until a friend told us 'he's not broken; stop trying to fix him.' That was the best advice anyone could have given us. Now instead of looking at age-appropriate charts, we celebrate all the small accomplishments he has. We continue to be proud of our son, given how hard he has to work to achieve the same end.

"I don't plan on looking at any more developmental charts unless it is to help decide on promotion to the next grade level or that kind of big decision."

—*Chris, mom to six-year-old James, autism (Syracuse, New York)*

in those rainbow-colored charts. It doesn't mean there's a problem; it just means it's a bit more complicated than organizing your sock drawer.

So you can let the boxes make you crazy. Or you can make the boxes your friend.

SPEECH AND LANGUAGE DEFINED

Think of speech as you would a toolbox filled with all the implements required to do the job—hammer, screwdriver, and so on. Language, on the other hand, is more like a beautifully handcrafted coffee table—the end result of using the tools to reach a goal.

Speech is the physical act of speaking; the oral expression of thoughts, feelings, ideas, and, when directed toward a toddler, often a directive not to drop the phone into the toilet. It's the result of precisely coordinated muscle actions in the head (including the mouth, jaw, tongue, and lips), neck, chest, and abdomen, and its development takes place gradually over years of practice. During this process, children learn how to use their muscles to produce understandable speech.

Language is what gives order to speech. It's basically a system of symbols—conventionally used signs, sounds, and gestures—that allow people to translate their thoughts, feelings, and ideas into messages that are understood within their community. If you're an English-speaking American traveling around Spain, you may have trouble communicating with the locals if you don't know Spanish—unless of course your Dora the Explorer–loving toddler can help you out.

But you don't have to leave the country to be aware of language differences between communities. For example, you might tell your best friend she looks *phat* in her new jeans if the two of you are hanging out at a hip hop club; it's unlikely you'd say the same to her at a Weight Watchers meeting.

A Breakdown in Communications, or Linguistics 101

Now that you understand the difference between speech and language, let's take a closer look at each.

Speech. Some of the factors that influence speech are:

- **Voice.** Pitch, loudness, and quality determine if your child's speech is adequate for communication and whether it suits her as an individual. If your four-year-old daughter sounds like Darth Vader or you can hear your nine-year-old son clear as a bell from ten rows away at a monster truck show, there might be a problem with their voice. Similarly, if you struggle to hear your daughter—even when she's sitting on your lap—or her voice sounds soft and breathy, this, too, may be a problem.
- **Prosody.** Prosody is the melody and rhythm of language; the emphasis we place on our words or the intonation of our speech. Your prosody varies depending on what you are talking about and to whom you are speaking. Most people, almost instinctively, use a high-pitched, sing-songy voice when talking to an infant. But

it's unlikely you'll use that same rhythm of speaking when you're making a presentation to a client.

- **Rate.** The speed—or lack thereof—with which your child speaks affects her ability to successfully communicate. She needs to talk slowly enough for others to follow along but fast enough that they don't lose interest. If listening to her reminds you of a bidding war at Sotheby's, she needs to slow down. If you keep checking your watch as she tells you what she had for lunch, she needs to pick up the pace.
- **Articulation.** Simply put, articulation is the ability to speak clearly and effectively. Not so simply put, it's what happens when sounds, syllables, and words are formed as a result of the tongue, jaw, teeth, lips, and palate working together and altering the air stream coming from the vocal folds. Some mispronunciation is developmental in nature and most children will come to articulate clearly over time. So if your two-year-old is requesting *pasketti* and meatballs for dinner, there's no need to worry—unless of course you're out of spaghetti.
- **Fluency.** Fluency is the natural flow of speech and something we take for granted until it is interrupted. Everyone has occasional moments of dysfluency; think back to the eighth grade . . . you probably weren't all that smooth the first time you talked with the cute guy from homeroom. Almost all children experience some developmental dysfluency—usually between two and five years old—that typically disappears as their communication skills evolve. Developmental dysfluency usually involves the repetition of whole words ("gum-gum") and phrases ("I want-I want"). Indications of a problem may be when the dysfluency turns into stuttering, which can take the form of an initial consonant repetition ("c-c-c-c-at") or prolongation of vowels ("c-aaaaaaaat") and may be accompanied by odd behaviors such as head slapping or eye blinking. Regardless, if the dysfluency begins to upset your child, occurs more frequently, or continues past age five, it's time to seek help.

Language. Language is also comprised of five distinct areas: phonology, morphology, syntax, semantics, and pragmatics. The terms may be new to you but trust me, you're already familiar with the concepts; you use them each and every time you talk, known as *expressive language*, as well as listen, which is *receptive language*.

- **Phonology.** Phonemes are individual speech sounds; phonology is the study of how these sounds fit together to make language. Kids learn, over time, which sounds go with other sounds to create words. For example, they know that their request for a pet *c*-at is more likely to be granted than a request for a pet *r*-at.
- **Morphology.** Morphology is the branch of grammar that studies the structure of words. All words are comprised of morphemes, which are the smallest grammatical unit of speech. Morphemes help us understand if your child is asking for one banana or a bunch of bananas. They tell us if you need to shop for bananas, if you've already shop*ped* for them, or, if your toddler fed the last one to your terrier, whether you'll be shop*ping* for more soon.
- **Syntax.** After you've used your phonemes to create morphemes, you'll need to know in what order to put them. That's where syntax comes in; it's the rules that determine how words are combined to create grammatical sentences. It's something children learn over time. Here's an example of typical sentence formation for different ages:

  18 months: "No bath me!"
  2 years: "Me no bath!"
  2½ years: "I no want bath!"
  3 years: "I don't want a bath!"

  Syntax doesn't make your kids any more cooperative, but it does help them protest in a more grammatically correct manner.

- **Semantics.** Semantics encompasses the words we know and use, but mainly, it has to do with the *meaning* of words and sentences. In a way, it's the meaning *behind* the words and sentences; it's how we interpret what someone intends, rather than the literal definition of the words she uses. For example, if your best friend told you her husband surprised her with a pair of diamond earrings, you might tell her, "I hate you." Will your friend be offended? Unlikely. Because she knows what you really mean is, "I wish my husband would surprise me with an extravagant gift."

- **Pragmatics.** For every conversation in which you nod in agreement, make eye contact, and wait your turn to talk, you are using your pragmatic language skills. Pragmatics refer to the social rules of communication, rules that most people don't consciously notice—until the person you're talking to breaks them—and they involve three different communication skills:

  1. *Using language for different purposes,* such as greeting, informing, demanding, promising, and requesting. That coworker who makes eye contact but never says hello when she passes you in the hall? She could use a little help with her social language.

  2. *Changing language based on the needs of the listener or the situation,* such as talking differently to a baby than to an adult, using different voices depending on your locale, or providing enough background information to an unfamiliar listener. So it's unlikely you would use baby talk with another adult or whisper at a rock concert. It's also why, when you're telling a friend about your latest job interview and an acquaintance joins the conversation, you fill her in on your idiot boss so she understands why you're looking for work.

  3. *Following rules for conversations,* such as introducing topics of conversation, staying on the topic, taking turns in conversation, rephrasing when misunderstood, and telling a story. There are also rules for nonverbal cues in conversation: distance between speaker and listener, facial expressions, and eye contact.

Now that you have an understanding of all the different components that impact speech and language, you can begin to see the different ways in which a child's communication can be impaired. Chapter 4 provides an overview of nine different types of disorders, but next, the importance of early intervention and why it's vital to detect a speech or language problem as early as possible. And now that you've been given an overview of typical language development, we'll follow up with the signs of not-so-typical development.

Oh, and just so you know . . . there's another chart coming your way.

2

Wait Is a Four-Letter Word: The Importance of Early Intervention

You'd think because I had already received a diagnosis for Max, studied everything about apraxia I could get my hands on, and spent two full years shuttling Max to and from speech therapy that when Ari started showing signs of a speech delay, I would be the last person to buy into what I consider to be the three most dangerous words one can say to a parent with concerns about her child: wait and see.

But I did.

My husband Dave and I first started to take note of Ari's speech when she was seventeen months old. According to the ubiquitous *What to Expect* books, she was on track, despite the fact that her three-word vocabulary of *mama*, *dada*, and *hi* seemed, to me, unusually small.

One month later, with the addition of *wow, all done, doggie*, and *pretzel*, her repertoire was up to eight words. Still not a lot, but it was the same number of words Max had when he was two and a half so I figured she was ahead of the game. She was ahead of where her brother had been, if nothing else.

By twenty months I was asking Jenny, Max's speech therapist, about getting Ari evaluated. She cautioned me that at Ari's young age it's harder to get accurate information, but that yes, she could be evaluated. In the meantime, she directed me to a developmental chart. According to this particular one, an 18–23-month-old was expected to:

- Use real words and fewer gestures when trying to get something (Ari used far more gestures.)
- Ask one- to two-word questions (She didn't.)
- Put two words together (No)
- Name one picture of a familiar object (Not any more)

I may have started out giving Ari the benefit of the doubt. But as more time passed I knew it was only a matter of time before we'd be given our second apraxia diagnosis. I just felt it. So I scheduled a meeting with Nancy Kaufman, the director of the speech center that had become—and it seemed, would continue to be—our second home. After the receptionist put me on the schedule, she handed me the standard parent questionnaires to fill out, and then removed one of the pages from the pile.

"I guess you don't need the map," she said.

Ari started therapy at twenty-two months but she wasn't officially given a diagnosis until a few months later, once her therapist could better assess her through their one-on-one sessions. She did, in fact, have apraxia.

Here's the point I want to make: I already had one child with a speech disorder. I was educated and informed. I was even in the middle of writing an article for one of the national parenting magazines on normal language development. I had half a dozen developmental charts on my desk and had been talking with top experts in the field. And *still*, I kept waiting and seeing. I guess I didn't want to presume Ari would follow in Max's verbal footsteps.

For some, waiting and seeing is easy. Waiting and seeing doesn't require any investment of emotional energy. Waiting and seeing doesn't call for you to fill out countless questionnaires and checklists and force you to look at your child under a microscope and speculate if something's wrong. Waiting and seeing is optimistic.

For others, waiting and seeing is difficult. It eats up your stomach lining. It makes you snap at your optimistic friends who insist nothing's wrong. It leaves you begging your doctor for an early referral. Waiting and seeing is grueling. Whatever our reason for waiting and seeing, too many of us are doing it.

The reasons why we sometimes wait to get our kids checked out are as different as our kids themselves. The overbearing grandmother who says you're worrying over nothing. The well-intentioned friend who reminds you—and she's the seventeenth person to do so—that Einstein didn't talk until he was three years old. The dismissive pediatrician. The spouse who argues that you're pushing your child too hard.

Maybe you're worried about the expense of therapy. (Don't be— free services are available. Check out Chapter 10.) Or you don't know where to go for help. (Check out Chapter 3.) Or you're afraid a formal evaluation might confirm your biggest fear, that there is in fact something wrong with your child. I know it's scary and overwhelming. I know it can feel like your world is turning upside-down—it did for me. Twice.

Here's what I want you to remember: *the sooner you get the answers, the sooner your child gets what she needs.*

It can also be hard to figure out *when* to seek help. It's like when you suspect your child has an ear infection; take him to the doctor too soon and there's nothing to detect. But take him too late and he's already in pain. The same holds true when you have a concern about your child's development; take him in too early and you might worry about being perceived as a neurotic parent. Take him in too late and learn your hunches were right, and you'll beat yourself up for not trusting yourself.

If you're not sure if it's time to be worried, the following chart can serve as a basic guideline for detecting atypical development. However, the most important sign you'll ever get isn't on any chart—it's that unsettled feeling in the pit of your stomach. Listen to it. It's right far more than it's wrong.

Troubling Speech and Language Development

It's time to consult a professional if:	Receptive Language	Expressive Language	Social Skills	Motor Skills
During the first 3 months your child:	Shows a lack of awareness of sound Shows a lack of awareness of her environment		Shows a lack of responsiveness to people	Has problems sucking or swallowing
From 3 to 6 months your child:	Doesn't localize the source of a sound or speaker Lacks an awareness of people and objects in the environment	Doesn't make cooing noises	Doesn't have a social smile Doesn't make eye contact Is easily overstimulated	
From 6 to 9 months your child:	Doesn't appear to understand or enjoy the social rewards of interaction	Doesn't take turns cooing with you Doesn't babble or babbles with few or no consonants	No longer uses cooing and babbling in interactions Doesn't make eye contact or makes less eye contact than at younger ages	
From 9 to 12 months your child:	Fails to give a toy to a parent whose hand is outstretched Only understands language that is accompanied by visual clues (For example, only understands	Vocalizes infrequently Focuses on an object of interest but doesn't make a clear request (verbal or gestural) Lacks consonants in vocalizations	May point, but only to express wants and needs; doesn't point to interesting objects or actions Doesn't attend to music or play with toys	Frequently gags or chokes on foods with new tastes or textures

	"time to put on shoes" if mom is holding shoes Doesn't understand verbal routines such as waving bye-bye Doesn't recognize her own name Doesn't look at parent in response to *mama* or *dada*	Lacks consistent patterns of reduplicative (dadadada or gagagaga, for example) babbling Lacks responses indicating comprehension of any verbal routines, words, or communicative gestures Doesn't imitate actions and familiar sounds	Is easily upset by sounds that would not be upsetting to others	
From 12 to 18 months your child:	Understands fewer than 50 words or phrases (without gestures or visual clues) Doesn't stop behavior when told "no"	Doesn't use words or add new words to a small vocabulary Loses most of her words she previously learned Speaks fewer than 10 words Doesn't try to imitate words she hears Doesn't babble sounds, especially *m, n, t, d, b, p,* and *z* sounds	Doesn't play pat-a-cake and peek-a-boo Doesn't look at what a parent is pointing out	Drools excessively (not related to new teeth)

(continued on next page)

Troubling Speech and Language Development (continued)

It's time to consult a professional if:	Receptive Language	Expressive Language	Social Skills	Motor Skills
From 18 to 24 months your child:	Has a reasonable, receptive vocabulary that is far larger than his expressive vocabulary Doesn't point to body parts on request Doesn't follow simple one-step commands ("Bring mama the book.")	Speaks fewer than 50 words Doesn't use any two-word combinations Relies on nonverbal gestures for communication Produces few consonant sounds Has largely unintelligible speech Tends to label objects instead of commenting or requesting Shows regression in language development or stops talking Uses pat phrases but does not create new phrases appropriate to the situation Begins echoing phrases he hears, often inappropriately	Doesn't regularly seek social interaction Doesn't engage in pretend play, such as feeding a doll or playing with trucks Tends to play by lining up toys or focusing on details such as the wheels of a car	
From 2 to 3 years your child:	Doesn't shake or nod her head in response to yes and no questions	Has more than 50 words but doesn't use any two-word combinations	Engages in brief pretend play with a single object (talking on the phone, feeding a baby) but cannot elaborate upon it	

From 3 to 4 years your child:	Demonstrates poor comprehension Doesn't understand concepts such as *big/little* and *one/all* Doesn't answer *what* and *where* questions Doesn't respond to two unrelated commands (*Give your sister the ball and come upstairs.*)	Uses only single syllable words with no final consonants Doesn't demand a response from listeners Doesn't ask questions Frequently tantrums when not understood Is only intelligible to family 50% of the time Continues to repeat what others say with no communicative intent	Only uses short, simple sentences Repeats individual sounds or shows other signs of stuttering Is only intelligible to strangers 50% of the time Doesn't effectively communicate with adults	Doesn't interact with peers for pretend play Doesn't take turns in conversation

(continued on next page)

Troubling Speech and Language Development (*continued*)

It's time to consult a professional if:	Receptive Language	Expressive Language	Social Skills	Motor Skills
From 3 to 4 years your child:		Has trouble expressing his ideas Doesn't ask *what* and *where* questions Doesn't sing familiar songs Talks incessantly about only one topic, such as animals or dinosaurs Uses flat, stilted, or unusual intonation		
From 4 to 5 years your child:		Makes errors in consonants such as *b, p, d, t, k, m, n, l, r, w, s* Doesn't effectively communicate with peers or strangers Doesn't count to five Doesn't name primary colors Doesn't answer simple questions such as *what, who, why,* and *how many?*	Doesn't share toys Doesn't use language in social interactions	

From 5 to 7 years your child:	Doesn't understand *between, above, below, top,* and *bottom*	Cannot recount the activities of the day or the usual sequence of common activities, such as taking a bath Doesn't tell familiar stories with picture cues Doesn't generate complex sentences (*I ate a peanut butter sandwich because I was hungry. We went to the zoo and saw monkeys.*) Doesn't use possessives consistently Isn't understood by familiar listeners most of the time Doesn't talk about her own feelings

Parent to Parent

I knew something was wrong when:

"At eighteen months my daughter Lauren had virtually no vocabulary. At twenty-four months she had less than twenty words and most often pointed, grunted, or screamed to get her wants and needs across. I knew that such a gross lack of language was not normal."

> —*Jean, mom to three-and-a-half-year-old Lauren, expressive and receptive speech and language impairment (Howell, Michigan)*

"At age two Alex still wasn't putting two words together. He had developed some simple language—'mommy up'—but then he seemed to lose it and we didn't know why."

> —*Cathy, mom to five-year-old Alex, high-functioning autism and apraxia (Elkins Park, Pennsylvania)*

"At age four my son was exhibiting mild first-word repetitions, which is common for all young children. But when he began hitting his stomach to force the first word out of his mouth, I became concerned. Also, my husband stutters, so he is acutely sensitive to any behavior that would indicate speech dysfluency."

> —*Kristen, mom to nine-year-old RJ, dysfluency (Trumbull, Connecticut)*

"Jordan's intelligibility of speech became a concern at about two and a half years old. She started to speak later than her sister and the speech was not as clear. At first it was kind of cute—'Garah' for her sister Sarah—but when it didn't show signs of clearing I became concerned."

> —*Sharon, mom to four-and-a-half-year-old Jordan, articulation disorder (Farmington Hills, Michigan)*

DELAY OR DISORDER?

I'm willing to bet you've been told, more than once, that nothing is wrong with your child and she's just a bit delayed. And she very well may be. She may be so focused on learning how to walk or developing her fine motor skills that communication has simply taken a temporary backseat. It may not matter that her brother or her cousins all started talking on the early side. Each child has her own timetable and some children will simply start talking long after their peers.

The difficulty lies in distinguishing between the kids who are delayed and the kids who have a disorder. Early on, this can be hard to do—even for a professional. Because speech and language are not a typical pediatrician's areas of expertise, he's not as likely as a speech-language pathologist to recommend testing, especially at a young age. It's likely he's thinking about that old medical adage that if you hear hoofbeats, think horses and not zebras. Some pediatricians still believe that a parent should wait until a child is two years old—or even three—before seeking an evaluation. They know that many children who are delayed at age two are closer to being developmentally on target by the time they turn three. They don't want to add to the parent's anxiety, so they wait to be sure there is in fact a problem. It's this kind of thinking that leads many parents to believe that it's OK to "wait and see" about their child's communication skills.

The reality is, with nearly three to six million children under the age of eighteen with speech and language disorders in the United States, there are far more zebras out there than your pediatrician may believe. Also, delays can persist and it can be unclear at which point to consider them a disorder.

So if you suspect a delay or a disorder, it's critical to have a qualified speech therapist make a diagnosis and suggest treatment if appropriate. Even if your child has only a simple delay, a good therapist will send you home with plenty of ideas on how to jump-start or improve your child's communication.

What exactly is a speech delay? Your child has a simple delay if his receptive and expressive language are coming along in an expected pattern of development but at a slower rate than average. His receptive and expressive skills are fairly even and he has the ability to catch up to his peers without the benefit of therapy.

A child with a speech disorder, however, doesn't have the same speech and language skills as his peers. He is not simply on the later side of normal development or a "late talker." He may have some age-appropriate skills but may be missing some of what should have been acquired at a younger age. There is something out of order or unusual about his speech or language and it won't resolve on its own. Disorders, much more so than delays, are likely to negatively impact a child's learning, behavior, and social development.

For example, a child who is delayed may acquire the ability to say vowel sounds, but at a slower rate than other children his age. A child who has a disorder may not acquire any vowel sounds, or they may be distorted. Here's another way to look at it: a three-month-old who takes turns cooing with you is developmentally on target. His two-year-old sister who can talk up a storm but doesn't respond to questions—that's a potential concern. A good rule of thumb is this: if the speech or language problem affects your child's functioning, either in learning or social interactions, then it's likely a disorder.

WHAT AFFECTS YOUR CHILD'S SPEECH AND LANGUAGE DEVELOPMENT?

There are many factors that play a role in your child's speech and language development. Some are behavioral characteristics that suggest whether or not a language-delayed child will catch up on her own or will require intervention. One researcher refers to these as *predictors of language change*. Basically, they're the little clues parents can keep tabs on to help measure just how worried we should be.

The other factors are those variables, either related to the family or behavior, that suggest a child is likely to have a true speech or language impairment rather than a delay. This same researcher calls these *risks*, and they're the elements of a child's particular situation that can change how she learns language.

A quick note before we explore predictors and risks—while the negative aspects of these factors can increase the risk of an actual problem, the mere presence of these factors doesn't indicate a problem. That said, here's a look at both in the sections that follow.

Predictors of Language Change

There are several predictors to look for:

Language Comprehension. Typically, your child will show an understanding of language long before she actually uses it herself. Some studies that followed up with late-talking children after a year found that those with true language delays did not have age-appropriate receptive language. The children who did were considered to simply be late bloomers. Additionally, for children who show a delay in both receptive and expressive language, the larger the gap between the two, the worse the outlook.

Use of Gestures. One study found that the number of gestures used by late-talking children with little expressive language can indicate later language abilities. Children with a greater number of communicative gestures (for example, pointing to the refrigerator to indicate hunger) are more likely to catch up with their peers. This is supported by findings that some older children who are taught nonverbal communication methods show a spontaneous increase in talking.

Researchers also found that late-talking children used more gestures to help communicate their wishes than those children whose speech was age-appropriate. However, this changes as children progress from using single words to two- and three-word phrases.

Typically developing children, for example, will shake their head while saying "no." (This is a complementary gesture.) The next step would entail the child shaking his head and saying "milk" to mean "no milk." (This is a supplementary gesture.) The expected evolution is the use of a single word alone, then a single word with a complementary gesture, followed by a single word paired with a supplementary gesture, and, finally, word combinations. The research found that children who don't follow this sequence of gesture use are appropriate candidates for speech therapy.

Age of Diagnosis. More than one study indicated that the older the child at the time of diagnosis, the less positive the outcome. Older children have had a longer time to develop than younger children but have not done so, indicating that the language delay may be more serious.

Progress in Language Development. Even if a child is slow in language development, she should still do new things with language at least every month, such as adding new words or using the same word for different purposes. For example, "doggie" may mean three different things on three different days: "I see a doggie." "That is my doggie." "Where is my doggie?" She should combine words into longer phrases ("doggie here" or "no doggie") and use them more often.

Language Production. The number of words your toddler has in his spoken vocabulary is a good reflection of his future language development. For example, a two-year-old with fewer than fifty words is considered at risk for continued delay—a risk that grows if the child continues to develop but his verbal repertoire doesn't.

The type of words he uses is also a factor; research has shown that children with speech and language impairments have little variation in the verbs they use, and tend to rely on general ones such as *want*, *go*, *put*, *look*, and *make*.

Phonology. How much does your baby babble? It matters more than you might think. Experts have found a correlation between prelinguistic vocalizations (otherwise known as babbling) and future language learning. Several studies found a relationship between the number of consonants in a toddler's babbling and his future vocabulary development. And children who were delayed in expressive language not only used fewer consonants, but were also less accurate in their pronunciation.

Imitation. Before you ever hear your child say "more juice," it's likely you'll have to say it a few times first. Because before he can say new words on his own, he'll need to practice them. He does that by listening to you and imitating what he hears. Researchers found that toddlers who don't imitate two-word combinations, even with prompting, are likely in need of speech therapy.

Play. How your little one plays may very well indicate how he'll learn language later on. Late talkers who used toys together in meaningful ways (combinatorial or thematic play), such as making music with a spoon and pot, or better yet, who used toys for make-believe scenarios (symbolic play) such as driving a toy truck to a parking garage or feeding a baby doll with pretend food, have a greater chance of catching up than those late talkers who primarily played by handling and grouping toys, such as lining up cars and organizing action figures.

Social Skills. Preschoolers with communication impairments are more likely to choose the teacher for a conversation partner than their fellow classmates. One study found that in addition to receptive and expressive language, socialization skills were also lower in children with delayed expressive speech; these kids are more likely to play with toys in unusual ways, have trouble sharing, and be disinterested in playing with their peers.

Otitis Media. Otitis media is an inflammation in the middle ear that is usually associated with fluid buildup, which may or may not be infected. As it's the most frequently diagnosed disease in infants and young children, you're likely already familiar with its acute form, with associated fever, ear pain, and sleepless nights. But it also comes in a quieter form, not necessarily accompanied by these symptoms.

When fluid is present in the ear there can be some hearing loss— typically, it's akin to a quiet conversation being reduced to a loud whisper. This is temporary and typically resolves as the fluid buildup does. However, otitis media tends to occur during the child's first few years of life—a critical time for speech and language development. So even a temporary hearing loss can theoretically have a negative impact on communication skills. The challenge is often made all the more difficult when a child has otitis media without infection. If there's no infection, there usually isn't any pain or fever—nothing to indicate to a parent that something is wrong. Weeks or months of precious language learning can go by before parents realize there's a problem.

That said, there is some disagreement among researchers regarding the relationship between otitis media and speech and language development. For one thing, it is difficult to estimate just how accurate the parents are in their recollections of their child's early history of infection. Even when medical records are consulted, they don't necessarily include relevant information such as whether or not fluid accompanied each episode of infection or if there was hearing loss; this makes it difficult to clearly establish the correlation between otitis media and communication development.

One study shows that children who had persistent fluid buildup during the first three years of life and had tympanostomy tubes promptly inserted—this is the surgical treatment that relieves the fluid buildup—showed no differences in their language development compared to children allowed to go on with fluid and without the surgery.

The American Academy of Pediatrics recommends a hearing test for children with prolonged otitis media. If the hearing is within normal range then surgery may not impact the child's communication. But if the hearing is mildly abnormal, a surgical option should be discussed.

Risks

There are a number of risks associated with speech and language disorders.

Heritability. Research has been fairly consistent in establishing that children with a parent or sibling who had language or learning difficulties are at an increased risk of language delay. While this is a risk we have little control over, it would be worth investigating whether certain types of environmental stimulation or therapy for children in such families would improve their odds of recovery, thus minimizing family history as a risk factor.

Parental Influence. The way we interact with our children has also been linked to language development, although the research isn't completely clear. However, it does indicate that parents who talk and play with their children often, follow their lead in conversation, engage them by pointing out items of interest in their surroundings, and use simplified language are more likely to encourage language use and development than parents who are less responsive and more controlling of the child's activities and conversation topics. The former style is more often found in parents with a higher level of education; it is not necessarily the norm in parents with a lower level of education and income, thus making socioeconomic status yet another risk factor.

How your child's other caregivers interact with him also plays a role, so bear that in mind when selecting a daycare facility or preschool.

Hearing Loss. Children with hearing loss are at a great risk of delay in both receptive and expressive communication skills. If not addressed early on, this can lead to learning problems, social isolation, and poor self-esteem.

Thanks to the Universal Newborn Hearing Screening, the number of infants being screened for hearing loss has increased over the years. But that doesn't take into account those children who suffer a loss at a later age.

Children with a hearing loss are often difficult to understand; they usually can't hear quiet speech sounds such as *s, sh, f, t,* and *k,* so they don't include them in their speech. They may not hear their own voice and may speak too loudly or not loudly enough. Their pitch may be too high, or they may sound as if they are mumbling because of poor inflection or an inappropriate rate of speech.

Although it's true that the younger a child is at the time of a hearing loss, the more it will impact his development, early identification and intervention can minimize that impact. And research indicates that children who receive intervention early on may be able to develop language equal to that of their hearing peers.

Cognitive, Neurological, or Developmental Diagnosis. Children with cognitive impairment, neurological conditions (hydrocephalus, stroke, and seizures), and autistic spectrum disorders (autistic disorder, pervasive developmental disorder—not otherwise specified, Asperger syndrome) have a laundry list of medical, developmental, and behavioral challenges—speech and language typically being one of them. Sometimes the initial observation of a child's communication difficulties leads to the diagnosis of a broader problem, rather than one limited to a speech or language disorder.

It's important for parents—and professionals—to keep this in mind. An eighteen-month-old who doesn't seek out other children to play with may have a speech disorder and need help expressing himself verbally—or he may be presenting autistic characteristics. *This is not to say that if your child is having speech or language difficulties you should fear the worst.* It's just yet another reason why early detection is crucial. And only through early intervention by the appropriate professional (more on who that is in Chapter 3) can you know what your child needs.

SPEECH AND LANGUAGE MYTHS

We don't always know what causes speech and language problems. But we know what *doesn't* cause them:

- **Being a boy.** Studies show that while preschool-age boys develop language more slowly than preschool-age girls, the lag is only one or two months. His language skills would have to be in the 25th percentile to be considered significantly delayed. For example, a fifteen-to-eighteen-month-old would have to be functioning at the level of an eleven-to-fourteen-month-old to be considered significantly delayed. However, any concern should be addressed, as boys are more likely than girls to develop a speech or language disorder.
- **Living in a bilingual household.** The same language milestones apply whether a child is learning one or two languages. However, when children are exposed to the second language they may go through what is called a "silent period," when they speak very little and focus on learning and understanding the new language. They are likely to mix vocabulary and grammar rules between the two languages. These are normal behaviors and are signs of a language difference, not a disorder.
- **Having a parent or older sibling who anticipates the child's every need.** Talking is the most effective way for a child to get what he wants. If he is capable of communicating on his own, he will. If he doesn't, he most likely can't.
- **Having an older sibling with a speech problem.** Whether it's in preschool or at the supermarket with mom, most kids are exposed to plenty of people who speak correctly. It's unlikely he'll model

his own speech on the one person he knows who doesn't speak well.

- **Being stubborn.** How many kids would ever choose screaming, head-banging, and ineffective nonverbal gestures over opening their mouths and talking? That's right. None.

- **Having a tongue-tie.** The lingual frenum is the thin, vertical fold of tissue that attaches the undersurface of the tongue to the floor of the mouth. A child who has a short frenum—also known as ankyloglossia—has reduced mobility of the tongue. While parents are sometimes advised to consider surgery, it's important to note that a tongue-tie doesn't necessarily impair speech. In fact, the frenum may be tight because the child is not using his tongue normally. A speech-language pathologist would need to take into account the range of tongue movements, the points of attachment, and the child's speech development before advising for or against surgery.

Other pieces of well-intentioned advice to ignore:

- **He'll outgrow the problem.** Some will. Some won't. How can you tell which way your child will go? You can't.

- **She's too young to be evaluated.** Hearing can be tested in infants. How well a child understands language, how she plays, and how she interacts with others can also be easily assessed—just don't expect testing methods to include paper and a pencil.

- **He's not talking, so his speech can't be evaluated.** His receptive language—what he understands—can be evaluated, as can his pre-speech behavior, such as nonverbal communication. An evaluation can also provide parents with suggestions on encouraging their child's speech development.

- **Wait until she starts school.** The research is clear: the earlier a child receives services, the better her prognosis—not just for speech and language but for her overall development. And while

Professional Opinion

"I would always advise early intervention. Yes, there are children out there who progress at a slower pace and end up catching up to their peers without a negative effect on their learning or development. But there are also those who do not get early intervention and begin to establish errors in their speech-language development that become embedded into the child's repertoire. I would rather err on the side of caution than face the alternative. It cannot hurt a child to get a jump-start, or gentle push, in any area of development."

—*Jennifer Hill, speech-language pathologist (Sylvan Lake, Michigan)*

"When it comes to therapy, earlier is better. Sammi came to me at three and a half with only two words. Vocalizing was a struggle. She made very good progress, but at her age we should have been working on sentences—not one- and two-syllable words. Logan came to me at seventeen months with oral motor and feeding issues. After nine months he was discharged. I believe if we had waited, the outcome would have been quite different.

"I would rather give a child therapy who 'grows out of it' than make a child suffer and not be able to communicate as one 'waits and sees.'"

—*Darci Truax, speech-language pathologist (Gillette, Wyoming)*

free services are available through public schools, you don't have to wait until your child is of school age to take advantage of them; there are free programs for children starting at birth.

BETTER TO PLAY IT SAFE

It's estimated that about half of two-year-olds with a speech or language delay will catch up by age three or four. However, it's difficult to know on which side of that coin toss your child will fall.

But even knowing that your child has just a simple delay shouldn't preclude you—or your pediatrician—from considering speech therapy. For some children, having a speech delay may only have a minimal impact on his interactions with others. But for many, a simple delay isn't so simple. If talking doesn't come easily, a child may be reluctant to interact with peers in a playgroup or preschool and he may withdraw. Other children who struggle to speak may show their frustration in ways you'd rather they didn't, such as biting other children, hitting, throwing toys, and screaming.

For me, it wasn't Max's shortage of words that gave me the most cause for concern; it was when he started banging his head against the floor and wall from sheer frustration that I realized we couldn't afford to "wait and see" any longer.

Why Some Pediatricians Suggest You Wait and See

They're Not Trained to Identify Speech and Language Disorders. It's safe to say that most parents think of their pediatrician as a guide to their child's health and well-being. Sure, you'll consult your friends for advice and you'll read the magazines and books. But it's likely that most parents, when it comes to medical and developmental concerns, will defer to the judgment and expertise of their pediatrician.

The unfortunate reality is that most general practice pediatricians or family physicians, those who provide routine primary care, treat colds and ear infections, and make sure immunizations are up to date, are simply not given proper training when it comes to communication disorders. Other physicians, including developmental-behavioral pediatricians, neurodevelopmental disability experts, and some pediatric neurologists are specifically trained to identify such disabilities. One study reports that sixteen of its twenty participants—all of whom were medical students and residents—received only five hours or less training in speech-language pathology. And the problem isn't limited to detecting speech and language impairments: of the 16 percent of children who have disabilities (including speech-language disorders, global cognitive impairment, learning disabilities, and emotional and behavioral issues), only 20–30 percent are identified before starting school.

According to Mark Simms, M.D., a child development expert and professor of pediatrics at Medical College of Wisconsin, the issue isn't a lack of information. "What we know is buried in the speech and language pathology literature," he says. "It needs to be carried over into what the pediatricians are reading."

One study found that pediatricians who had periodic contact with speech-language pathologists had higher referral rates, suggesting, as Simms does, that if there were more of a crossover, fewer children would slip through the cracks.

Mild Delays Are Difficult to Detect. While there is general agreement among medical professionals as to what constitutes a clear-cut delay, there isn't a consensus on determining at what point evaluation and intervention are necessary. This is because kids develop in spurts, making mild delays difficult to detect and interpret.

That said, it's interesting to note the results of a study that asked medical students and residents, and speech-language pathologists, to determine if referrals were necessary based on different scenarios. One hundred percent of the speech-language pathologists (SLPs) made referrals for apraxia of speech and stuttering, compared to 71 percent and 86 percent, respectively, of the medical student/resident group. The students and residents again fell short when only 24 percent of them referred for voice disorder compared to 95 percent of the speech therapists. It's statistics such as these that make it clear that medical schools need to evaluate how well they're preparing their students. And it's one more reason why parents need to follow their instincts—and not solely rely on their pediatrician's recommendations.

They Don't Conduct Screenings. According to a survey conducted by the American Academy of Pediatrics (AAP), 94 percent of respondents agreed that pediatricians should ask about a child's development. However, when it came to actually conducting developmental assessments, or screenings, 80 percent cited time limitation as a barrier. Fifty-five percent felt restricted by inadequate reimbursement from insurance companies. And 46 percent claimed "unfamiliarity with CPT codes" as a reason for not doing developmental assessments. Know what a CPT code is? It's one of those numbers on the piece of paper you take up front to cash out at your doctor's office; each medical procedure is assigned one.

For a doctor to not conduct a developmental assessment because she doesn't understand which code to use would be like you not submitting your tax return for a refund because you couldn't find a stamp. It's a poor excuse.

Granted, there are problems associated with pediatricians administering speech and language tests (aside from the ones cited in the AAP survey): they're simply not trained to administer them. So the tests are "dumbed down," according to Simms, so anyone can give them, and by doing so something is lost in the process.

Simms believes pediatricians shouldn't focus on screenings, which are specific tests that require time to administer and score, as well as a thorough understanding of speech and language development and disorders. Instead they should be relying more on surveillance—observing and interacting with the child during visits, asking parents about their concerns, and tracking development over time.

In 2006, noting that "early identification of developmental disorders is critical to the well-being of children and their families," the American Academy of Pediatrics issued a policy statement recommending developmental surveillance be incorporated at every well-child preventive care visit, and screening tests be administered regularly at the nine-, eighteen-, and thirty-month visits. This is hopefully a step in the right direction.

But the key is for pediatricians to know what typical and atypical development look like. "The screening tool should be your brain," Simms insists. "The most important part of the stethoscope is what's between the earpieces. The tool is the crutch, and if you don't have the knowledge and experience the tool won't work."

They Don't Know Where to Refer You. Think it's confusing trying to figure out where to go for help? Guess what . . . your pediatrician feels the same. According to the AAP, 46 percent of pediatricians surveyed said their lack of understanding of the early intervention program's processes and procedures was a barrier to referring children three years old and younger. And unless they are informed as to the private facilities offering speech services, you're left to find those on your own.

They're Afraid of Making You Anxious. It's ridiculous, I know. But according to a policy statement issued by the American Academy of Pediatricians, some pediatricians who screen patients find it a problem when they identify a child who requires a thorough evaluation for developmental disabilities because of the anxiety it inevitably provokes in parents. This concern may create a tendency for doctors to identify only markedly delayed children—which puts those children with milder delays at risk of not being evaluated, and possibly treated, at the earliest opportunity.

They Already Think You're Overly Anxious. Who of us hasn't, at some point, called our pediatrician because we thought our child was sleeping or eating or peeing or pooping too much? Or too little? It's in our job description as parents to worry about our kids, even if it means we also worry that the doctor thinks we're worrying too much. A good pediatrician will always encourage you to call with questions—and won't make you feel like your concerns are unfounded or silly.

Because they are not trained to detect speech and language irregularities, many doctors will suggest you wait and see—especially if your child's delays aren't significant. They may think you are worrying over nothing and may not take your concerns seriously.

The fact is, studies show that a parent's report of his child's skills is predictive of developmental delay. And parent concerns about speech and language were highly accurate for identifying the majority of children with true problems.

Why You Shouldn't Wait and See

Neuroplasticity Is at Work. The first three years of your child's life is a critical period as the rate of learning and development is most rapid at this time. (Kind of explains all those foreign language DVDs and classical music CDs marketed to the little ones.) While the human brain will change throughout a lifetime as it processes new information—this is called neuroplasticity—it is during the early years that rapid changes take place and this is why early intervention is so important. If a child is not learning how to communicate when he, or rather, his brain, is most ready, there's the risk he may have a harder time learning this skill at a later age.

One report showed that children with disabilities who received early intervention services showed significant developmental improvement after only one year. And according to the American Academy of Pediatrics, it is especially important to recognize delays in language skills early because early intervention may improve the prognosis of children with hearing loss and may enable earlier diagnosis of cognitive impairments and pervasive developmental disorders. Waiting until a young child misses a major milestone may result in late rather than early recognition.

Improved Family Well-Being. When a speech or language problem goes undetected, there's much more at risk than just the child's communication development. Children with developmental delays are at a higher risk for behavioral problems, and parents need strategies for getting through the day-to-day frustrations of living with a child with limited communication skills.

It's common for parents to feel disappointment, social isolation, added stress, frustration, and helplessness. I know I spent that first month after Max's apraxia diagnosis, in and out of tears—and being at my desk at work did nothing to stop the flow. Not surprising, parents of special needs kids are also at greater risk of divorce.

But with early detection and treatment, the negative impact of the child's disability is lessened. You have a game plan to follow. The child's frustration level is decreased because he is better able to communicate. And once the parents have an understanding of their child's disorder, they are better equipped to help him—and dedicate more time to family activities, focus on work, and be in a better position to support each other during a stressful time. I know that once Max started to develop language, he had fewer outbursts, he slept better, and my husband and I were able to do simple things with him that were previously unimaginable, such as spending time at the mall or eating in a restaurant.

Benefits Beyond Your Family. Research has shown that children who participate in early intervention programs require fewer special education services later in life, are held back a school grade less often, and, in some cases, are indistinguishable from nondisabled classmates years after intervention. The developmental and educational progress they make means a decreased dependence on support services and, in the long run, increased eligibility for employment—all of which provides economic and societal benefits.

Whether you came to this book with the knowledge that something was wrong with your child's communication or you needed to know whether or not to listen to your suspicions, I hope this information will help you move forward in getting your child checked out. (And get anyone in your life who isn't taking the issue seriously to get on board.) "But where do I start?" you may be asking. The next chapter will discuss the different professionals you can turn to for help.

3

Diving into the Alphabet Soup: Deciphering the M.D.s, Ph.D.s, and SLPs to Find the Right Expert for Your Child

I didn't get it right the first time.

Max was twenty-two months when we started speech therapy at a facility recommended by our pediatrician. The therapist was young and energetic and had a room full of toys in which to engage Max and, hopefully, elicit some speech. After five months, there was still no improvement. I chalked it up to Max's stubborn personality and decided to take a break from therapy. It wasn't until a few months later, when Max was diagnosed with apraxia—by another therapist, that I realized Max's lack of progress had nothing to do with his temperament. Once I understood the diagnosis and what was required, I realized that his speech pathologist had been using inappropriate techniques; Max never would have made any progress with her.

Max was correctly diagnosed by therapist number two—over the phone. Gail Gallante was a speech therapist in New York. We were in Michigan. My cousin Rachel knew we would be coming to New York to celebrate Thanksgiving with my family and strongly encouraged us to make an appointment with Gail, who was working with Rachel's daughter. At first I resisted. It seemed silly to go out of state for an evaluation. But then I figured we were going to be there anyway, Gail was being recommended by someone I trusted, and I knew I'd get an honest assessment because Gail had nothing to gain beyond the initial evaluation fee; she could have recommended ten speech sessions a week—it wasn't as if we would be flying in from Michigan to see her for therapy.

I called Gail to make an appointment and I filled her in on Max: his vocabulary of about six words, pointing, grunting, and screaming as his main forms of communication, his refusal to imitate, the increase in head banging.

"Sounds like apraxia," she said.

A few weeks later, after spending more than two hours with Max, Gail confirmed this diagnosis.

When we returned to Michigan I knew I had to find a therapist familiar with apraxia. I first contacted our state's early intervention program, and after therapist number three met with Max, she agreed that he required therapy. But she was only willing to see Max two days a week—not the four days Gail insisted was necessary if Max was going to start talking. I knew we would have to find a private therapist to supplement the early intervention services.

I remembered that my friend Meredith had a friend who was a speech therapist and asked for her number. Jennifer Hill, therapist number four, turned out to be the angel who finally helped Max find his voice.

I share this with you not to add to your frustration or feelings of being overwhelmed, but to point out that it may take more than one evaluation or one professional to find the correct answer to your child's difficulties. If your child is having other issues in addition to speech, whether it's physical, emotional, or social, you'll most likely need the services of a neurologist, developmental-behavioral pediatrician, or psychologist in addition to those of a speech-language pathologist. There is no right or wrong way to proceed—the most important thing is that you get started.

This chapter will review the different medical professionals you may come across while having your child assessed or treated. It's meant to give you an idea of what each specialist does and how he or she can best serve your child's needs.

While many parents tend to start with their pediatrician—and I encourage you to do this—you'll see that this chapter, however, does not. Far too many parents are given the "don't worry" line by pediatricians, and their search for information ends before it begins.

That the review of professionals in this chapter begins with the speech therapist—and not the pediatrician—is quite deliberate. It's important to know that you are free to consult with a speech therapist at any time, with or without a referral from your pediatrician. (If the referral is required for insurance purposes you can always seek a free evaluation through early intervention. Or, you can consult a different doctor.) You know your child better than anyone—including the folks with the M.D.s after their names—so that puts *you* in charge of your child's care.

Whether you are starting, or continuing, your journey, know that you will come across different professionals with varying degrees of experience and expertise. The most important thing to remember is the expertise you bring—as your child's parent and advocate. If a doctor or therapist offers an explanation that doesn't make sense to you, find another professional. Keep asking questions until you find one who is not only knowledgeable and compassionate, but also recognizes the importance of your involvement.

THE SPEECH-LANGUAGE PATHOLOGIST

A licensed speech-language pathologist (SLP), also known as a speech therapist, holds a master's degree in speech pathology (some may have a Ph.D.) as well as certification through the American Speech-Language-Hearing Association (ASHA). It is the SLP's job to assess, diagnose, and treat a broad range of speech and language difficulties. A speech therapist works with a wide range of children and difficulties—everything from the child with mild articulation problems to the child with autism who needs help in learning the social aspects of language, such as turn taking in conversation and staying on topic.

The SLP will need a thorough medical, social, and developmental history of your child, so expect to fill out several different questionnaires and checklists about his developmental milestones. Depending on how she prefers to work, the therapist may use informal methods of testing your child, formal assessments, or a combination of both during your first consultation.

If she's using informal methods, it may seem as if all she's doing is playing with your child, but between the bubble blowing, puzzle piecing, coloring, and role playing with Barbie and Darth Vader (a good SLP will be stocked with a complete arsenal of children's favorites), she's developing a rapport with your child, gaining his trust and evaluating several things:

- **His receptive language.** How well does your child attend to, process, understand, retain, and integrate spoken language?
- **His expressive language.** How easily can he put words together to formulate his thoughts and express them verbally?
- **His oral motor function.** Are his tongue, lips, jaw, and facial muscles working together to formulate words? Are there any physical abnormalities? Does he have trouble chewing, sucking, and blowing?
- **His body positioning.** How is his overall muscle tone and breath support, and are they impacting his speech?
- **His behavior.** Is the SLP able to engage him in play? Does he respond appropriately to exciting toys? Is his behavior similar to that of his peers?

At the end of your appointment, she'll give you her impressions and possibly a diagnosis. I say possibly because often the SLP will need to work with a child for a length of time to more precisely determine the exact cause of the problem. She'll advise you on what kind of therapy would best serve your child and how often he'll need it. You should also receive a written evaluation in the coming weeks.

Where to Find an SLP

You can always search ASHA's online database (asha.org) for a licensed therapist in your area. Or ask a friend or doctor for a recommendation. It shouldn't be too difficult to find one, as SLPs work in a wide range of settings.

University Clinic

- **Pro:** If the university's primary goal is to provide its students with a training ground, your fees will be extremely low. For two hour-long sessions a week, one mom paid only $150 for the entire semester. (That's compared to upwards of $100 an hour for private services.) Therapy is conducted by students, so you can hopefully expect to work with someone who is energetic, eager, and motivated to best serve your child. Since students are closely supervised by experienced SLPs, you have the added benefit of multiple opinions. Universities hire well-respected professionals whose performances are monitored through annual reviews.
- **Con:** Not all university speech clinics offer reduced fees, so you may end up paying the same amount of money as you would to a private therapist. Which is fine, except that you'll most likely be working with a student therapist who hasn't yet earned her degree or certification. The students are always closely supervised by a seasoned SLP, so the quality of the services will depend on the student, the supervisor, and how well they collaborate on what your child needs. The students often rotate off a case once their course of study is completed, whether or not your child has completed his therapy. If your child is severely impaired or has multiple diagnoses, he may be better served by working directly with an experienced therapist.

Parent to Parent

"The student therapist needed quite a bit of direction, but the clinical coordinator was always there to help. What was great for us is that the students are not set in their ways and are willing to try almost anything. They used the speech therapy model based on Stanley Greenspan's Floortime. No early intervention therapist would have done that with him."
—*Kelly, mom to five-year-old Payton, receptive and expressive delay, semantic and pragmatic language issues (Milwaukee, Wisconsin)*

Hospital Outpatient Clinic

- **Pro:** If the hospital accepts your insurance, you may be spared the administrative nightmare of submitting expenses and fighting rejected payments. If your child has additional medical needs or requires services such as occupational or physical therapy, a hospital setting can offer the ease of one-stop shopping. As with a university clinic, there are high standards when it comes to hiring therapists.

- **Con:** Whether or not the speech clinic is in a medical office building or the hospital itself, some parents may be put off by a hospital setting, where their child is a "patient" rather than a "client." Depending on the set-up, you may or may not be able to observe your child's sessions. And while it's potentially advantageous from an insurance standpoint, once your approved number of sessions are used, you'll need to pay out of pocket. This is true of any speech facility, but hospital fees may be higher than that of a private speech center because the overhead costs are higher.

Private Facility

- **Pro:** A private facility will offer you the most flexibility and very personalized service. Unlike some early intervention therapists who have to double or triple up their sessions because of heavy caseloads, private therapy offers one-on-one therapy, specifically designed to work on your child's particular issues. You can find specialists who have expertise in a particular diagnosis that may require a certain therapeutic approach. The facility is likely to be set up with one-way mirrors so you can observe your child's session and apply what is being done in therapy back at home. You and the therapist decide together how long the sessions will be and how many per week are necessary based on your child's needs. Service is continuous because they're not following a school calendar. Children who are turned down by early intervention programs can be serviced privately. And if you feel the therapist isn't connecting with your child or doesn't have the right experience, you can always try someone else.

- **Con:** Compared to the free services offered through early intervention programs, private speech therapy is expensive, with some therapists receiving upwards of $100 per hour. Multiply that by the two, three, or four sessions per week some children require and you're looking at a high monthly bill that may or may not be covered by insurance.

Early Intervention and Special Education Services

- **Pro:** Under the federal Individuals with Disabilities Education Act (IDEA), children with disabilities, including those with speech and language impairments, are eligible for special services from birth up to age twenty-two. (The early intervention system is for children from birth to three years; special education applies to those age three through twenty-two.) Should your child qualify for services, he'll receive speech therapy—for free. You'll work with a coordinator who, in addition to setting up a speech evaluation with an SLP, can also determine if your child should be assessed in any other areas, such as fine and gross motor skills, social skills, and emotional and behavioral development. If he requires help in any of these areas, the coordinator will make the appropriate arrangements for your child to be seen by an occupational therapist, psychologist, or another professional—also free of charge. Once your child's needs are assessed, appropriate goals will be made and written into either an Individualized Family Service Plan (IFSP) or Individualized Education Plan (IEP), depending on his age. Both are documents that spell out what services or accommodations your child needs in order to receive a free appropriate public education (FAPE). School-age children can receive speech services either right before, after, or in the middle of their school day, making the logistics of transportation and getting time off work much easier for the parent.

- **Con:** Although early intervention services are free, there's far less flexibility overall compared with private services. Although programs may vary a bit from state to state, it's likely that when school is out of session, your child is out of speech therapy. Con-

"My son started to talk, around age three, due to early intervention services. My daughter never got early intervention—we adopted her at a later age than we adopted my son—and she went right into special education. I feel firmly that if she had been having speech services from an early age she would not have speech and language problems at all."
—*Terri, adoptive mom to sixteen-year-old Elena, language-based learning disorders and thirteen-year-old Andrew, fetal alcohol effects (Clifton, New Jersey)*

tinuity is essential for successful therapy, so unless you can afford to supplement with private services, he'll have gaps in his therapy over summer and holiday breaks. The criteria used to determine if your child qualifies for services are much more stringent than in private practice, so many parents are told their child doesn't qualify—which may mislead them to believe that their child doesn't need speech therapy. The child very well may; he just doesn't meet the program's criteria. If he does qualify, you may or may not have a say in which speech therapist he'll see. Again, this depends on how the program runs in your state. Heavy caseloads mean fewer one-on-one sessions and more group speech therapy—which may or may not be the right thing for your child—and possibly not enough sessions per week. If services are offered at a school location, it's unlikely you'll be able to observe the sessions. And if your child is pulled from class in the middle of the day for speech, you and the therapist will have to make a more concerted effort to talk about your child's progress.

When to See an SLP

Make an appointment with an SLP if your child shows any of the warning signs from the chart in Chapter 2 (see page 24); you have no other concerns about his other areas of development; you want to get an idea of what free services your child is eligible for before paying for private services; or you'd like to supplement your private therapy.

THE AUDIOLOGIST

Talking and hearing are so interrelated that you'd be hard pressed to find a doctor or speech therapist who doesn't recommend you see an audiologist, just as a precaution. Even if you're confident that your child's hearing is not the issue, it's a quick, easy, and painless appointment that leaves you with one less unknown factor in determining your child's speech difficulties.

Audiologists diagnose and treat children and adults with hearing loss. (Balance problems, too.) He'll ask you about your child's medical history—number of ear infections, medications she may be taking, health conditions—as well as the pregnancy and delivery. He'll examine your child's ears to make sure there aren't any structural irregularities, excessive earwax, or a hole in the eardrum. And depending on your child's age, he'll rely on a number of tests to gather detailed information about whether your child can hear different sounds—low pitch, high pitch, loud, soft—as well as check for fluid in the middle ear, or other abnormalities, that can affect hearing. If your child has a hearing problem, the audiologist will fit her with hearing aids and monitor her improvement.

Where to Find an Audiologist

You'll find audiologists working in hospitals, medical centers, universities, or in private practice, either independently or in affiliation with a speech therapy facility or ear, nose, and throat physician. If you're having trouble getting a recommendation, you can search through the websites of the American Academy of Audiology

(audiology.org) or the American Speech-Language-Hearing Association (asha.org).

When to See an Audiologist

Make an appointment with an audiologist if your child doesn't seem aware of sounds around her, doesn't understand simple phrases such as "wave bye-bye," or she doesn't hear you when calling her name. (It doesn't count if she's watching TV.) If you're not worried about her hearing but have concerns about her speech or language, getting her hearing tested really is considered standard protocol.

YOUR PEDIATRICIAN

Pediatricians, as well as family practitioners, are encouraged by their professional organizations to provide what is referred to as a "medical home" for all children. The medical home is not a physical location, but rather an approach to providing comprehensive care. It's a service that's especially appealing to parents of children with developmental delays, disorders, or other chronic conditions. The physician is available to help parents find answers to their questions—which may involve a referral to one of the specialists discussed here. She'll direct you towards the appropriate resources and services, serve as coordinator of all the information you'll gather from other professionals, and give you whatever support you may need in determining the best course of action for your child.

In all likelihood, you already have a pediatrician; whether or not you feel she's taking your concerns seriously or is providing the support and services you need is another matter. If you're looking for someone who can, in addition to treating your child, serve as coordinator of the various professionals involved, you can search the database of the American Academy of Pediatrics (aap.org) or visit the National Center of Medical Home Initiatives for Children with Special Needs (medicalhomeinfo.org) for more information. Of course, word of mouth is often the best way to find an exceptional pediatric practice.

It's always best to start with your pediatrician because, unless your child has another medical condition, she's the one professional who knows your child the best. She can recommend specialists and serve as coordinator of all the information you're bound to come across.

Either you or your pediatrician may conclude that your child would benefit from a visit with a specialist. In the sections that follow are whom you're most likely to consult.

THE DEVELOPMENTAL-BEHAVIORAL PEDIATRICIAN

A general practice pediatrician can treat your child from top to bottom—literally, from cradle cap to diaper rash—and she can help manage kids with chronic conditions. A developmental-behavioral pediatrician (a DBP from here on out), however, has additional training in child development and specializes in treating children with developmental delays, disorders, and behavioral concerns.

During your visit, she'll assess your child's development in several areas: muscle tone, movement, language, fine and gross motor skills, and play behavior. Once she determines the nature of your child's difficulties, she can then refer you to any necessary specialists as well as serve as coordinator. If your child's difficulties aren't limited to speech and language, you're likely to have several experts in your employ (for example, an occupational therapist if he has sensory issues or a psychologist if behavior is a problem), and you may need a DBP to help you wade through all the options to decide the best course of treatment.

Where to Find a Developmental-Behavioral Pediatrician

Your best bet is always to get a recommendation from another parent or your doctor. Don't be afraid to ask your regular pediatrician for a name—if she's doing her job, she'll recognize that your child requires the care of a specialist and she'll make the referral before you even have to ask. If you're not comfortable, or come up short, the American Academy of Pediatrics (aap.org) has an online database you can search by state and specialty. Any children's hospital should also be able to refer you to this specialist.

When to See a Developmental-Behavioral Pediatrician

Consider seeing a developmental pediatrician when you, and/or your regular pediatrician need help in understanding and managing your child's problems; if your child has been diagnosed with a developmental, behavioral, or serious medical disorder such as cerebral palsy, ADHD, autism, fetal alcohol syndrome, or cognitive impairment; or if your child shows motor or cognitive delays in addition to a language delay.

THE PEDIATRIC OTOLARYNGOLOGIST

Also known as ear, nose, and throat (ENT) doctors, these specialists help patients with disorders and diseases of the ear, nose, and throat—as well as related structures of the head and neck. They are trained in both the medical and surgical treatment of a range of problems that can play a role in your child's speech and language development: hearing problems, ear infections, tinnitus (ringing in the ears), congenital disorders of the ear, diseases of the larynx (voice box) and esophagus, as well as voice disorders.

Where to Find a Pediatric Otolaryngologist

The best strategy is to get a referral from your pediatrician, who likely has a relationship with the specialists in your area and can make a recommendation, or visit the American Academy of Otolaryngology—Head and Neck Surgery (entnet.org) website and search the database. You can also contact your local hospital for a list of practitioners in your area.

When to See a Pediatric Otolaryngologist

Consider a visit with a pediatric otolaryngologist if you suspect your child has a hearing loss or possible voice disorder; if he's already been diagnosed with a cleft lip and palate or Down syndrome; or has any other condition that is likely to affect his ears, nose, or throat.

THE PEDIATRIC NEUROLOGIST

Neurologists specialize in diagnosing and treating disorders of the nervous system, which includes the brain, spinal cord, muscles, and nerves. After taking your child's medical history, the neurologist will check his coordination, strength, and reflexes by having him do such simple movements as squeezing her hand and balancing on one foot. And she'll screen for developmental problems, such as delayed motor skills or speech.

Where to Find a Pediatric Neurologist

Your pediatrician should be able to refer you to a pediatric specialist; if not, the American Academy of Neurology (aan.com) has a searchable online database. Or call your local hospital for a list of private practice neurologists.

When to See a Pediatric Neurologist

Make an appointment with a pediatric neurologist if you notice that your child is having staring episodes, unusual movements, uneven use of the two sides of his body, extreme muscle weakness, or he's complaining of headaches; or if your child has already been diagnosed with a seizure disorder, tic disorder, cognitive impairment, or hydrocephalus.

THE PEDIATRIC PSYCHOLOGIST OR PSYCHIATRIST

Because speech and language issues may be symptomatic of a broader problem—autism, for example—you may require the services of a mental health professional. Both the pediatric psychologist and psychiatrist will evaluate your child's problem by looking at him through a variety of lenses—developmental, emotional, cognitive, educational, and social. The psychiatrist, who holds an M.D., will also look at any physical or genetic components that may factor in to your child's difficulties. Both will ask you about your concerns, as well as take a medical history—yours and your spouse's as well as your child's. Depending on your child's age, she may involve him during your initial assessment by talking, drawing pictures, or playing with toys. Don't be surprised if you're only given a tentative diagnosis or first impression—it often takes several interactions with your child, and sometimes formal diagnostic testing, to reach an accurate diagnosis.

Where to Find a Pediatric Psychologist or Psychiatrist

Personal references are always best, so start by asking friends, your pediatrician, or even one of your own doctors. Your area hospital can refer you to either a psychologist or psychiatrist or, if there's one in your area, try a university clinic. The American Psychological Association has a searchable database at apahelpcenter.org.

When to See a Pediatric Psychologist or Psychiatrist

Consider a pediatric psychologist or psychiatrist if your child is having behavior problems, excessive anxiety, sensory issues, explosive fits, or is having trouble playing with other kids; or if you notice odd behaviors such as excessive twirling, mimicking, or an obsessive fascination with something not typically of interest to a child, such as maps or fans.

I know how difficult it is when you realize that your child is struggling with something. And finding the right professional to help your child can be overwhelming and equally stressful; hopefully, you now feel a little more prepared as you begin your search.

In the next chapter we'll explain nine different speech and language disorders—what causes them, what characteristics you should look for, how they may affect your child, as well as conditions that often coexist with speech and language impairment.

4

Learning the Lingo: Becoming Fluent in the Language of Speech and Language Problems

Personally, I like labels.

Whether it's a red and white one on a can of soup or a diagnosis being applied to one of my kids, labels give me valuable information. Am I about to ingest a mere one hundred calories—or a whopping five hundred? Is there enough protein in it to get me through until dinner? Is his communication problem receptive or expressive? Mild, moderate, or severe? How long until it's heated? Until he's fixed?

Labels help us understand what's inside—whether we're talking ingredients or diagnostic criteria. They help us put into words all the concerns we've had but perhaps were unable to intelligently articulate. Because while it's easy to see when our children don't communicate or behave as their peers do, it's not always so easy to understand why. And without labels, how in the world would we know what to Google?

What follows is a breakdown of children's speech and language disorders. Whether you're trying to figure out if your child has an actual disorder or you know she does and you're looking for easy-to-understand information on a diagnosis you've already been given, this chapter will prove useful. Of course, it can never take the place of a full evaluation by a licensed speech-language pathologist.

But then, nothing can take the place of an informed parent, either.

SPEECH AND LANGUAGE DISORDERS

Apraxia

May also be referred to as childhood apraxia of speech, developmental apraxia, verbal dyspraxia.

What Is It? Apraxia is a presumably neurological speech disorder that affects a child's ability to plan, execute, and sequence the precise series of movements of the tongue, jaw, lips, and palate that are necessary for intelligible speech. This is known as verbal apraxia. Oral apraxia, by contrast, is used to describe difficulty with nonspeech movements such as blowing, puckering, and licking food from the lips. Children with verbal apraxia are able to hear and understand words; but they have trouble with the motor skill necessary for formulating consonants and vowels into spoken words. While they may have a few words or phrases that they can speak clearly—what's referred to as "pop-outs"—they are unable to imitate what is asked of them.

What Causes It? While researchers have several theories, the cause of apraxia is not yet known. Some believe it is the result of an auditory or hearing deficit that affects the child's ability to detect and/or encode speech sounds from conversational speech. Others suggest apraxia is a language-learning problem; that the child has trouble producing speech because of his difficulties building an adult-like language system. One theory proposes that children with apraxia can store sounds and syllables in their brains but lack the ability to consistently organize and sequence the necessary movements in order to produce intelligible speech. And there are those who feel that apraxia is a neurological disorder that affects the brain's ability to send the proper signals to move the muscles involved in speech. Researchers in England have identified a gene within one family that has been linked to apraxia. However, it's unlikely that this gene is responsible for the majority of children with the disorder.

What Are the Signs?

Early on, children may have a very hard time learning their first words:

- Limited or little babbling as an infant
- First words may never appear; pointing and grunting may be all that is heard
- Grunting and pointing are primary methods of communication beyond age two
- First word approximations occur past eighteen months without developing into understandable words by age two
- One word or phrase is used in place of other words beyond age two

As children get older and learn some language skills, the problems become far more specific:

- May say words or phrases clearly on occasion but are unable to repeat or imitate when asked
- Consonant errors in conversational speech are highly variable (for example, a child may correctly say "baby" and the next time pronounce it "naby")
- Vowel errors in conversational speech are highly variable (for example, a child may correctly say "dog" and the next time pronounce it "dug")
- Limited consonant use; child may only use b, m, p, t, d, and h.
- May struggle with word retrieval issues, that is, locating and articulating the appropriate word.
- Significant discrepancy between what child understands (receptive language) and what he can articulate (expressive language)

- Spoken words are simplified by leaving out sounds or replacing them with sounds that are easier to say ("train track" becomes "tai tak")
- Variability in speech errors ("hat" may be pronounced as "hut," "ha," or "hu")
- Can say single words clearly but becomes unintelligible as sentences become longer

How Is It Treated? Children with apraxia require frequent and intensive one-on-one therapy in order to make speech automatic. The speech-language pathologist (SLP) will engage your child with a lot of repetition of sounds, starting with syllables and then progressing to words and sentences, to improve the muscle coordination and sequencing necessary for speech. She'll use visual and tactile cues to help him learn what his lips, tongue, and jaw look and feel like when making specific sounds.

Articulation Disorders

What Is It? Articulation is the way in which a child produces a sound and the placement of the tongue, lips, and teeth. A child with an articulation disorder has trouble with the physical production of individual speech sounds and may substitute, omit, or distort particular sounds. The term can be used generally for any problem with pronunciation, or more specifically for speech sound disorders

Parent to Parent

"Jordan used 'back' sounds for 'front' ones. She would say 'gog' instead of dog and 'Garah' for her sister Sarah."
    —*Sharon, mom to four-and-a-half-year-old Jordan, articulation disorder (Farmington Hills, Michigan)*

that may occur within individual sounds or within words. Common examples of articulation problems are lisps, immature pronunciation of r's, and substituting y for l.

What Causes It? For many kids, there may not be a clear explanation for an articulation disorder. For some, the cause can be due to neurological impairment, a cleft palate, or other physical abnormality, hearing loss, or brain damage.

What Are the Signs?
- Sound omissions ("bu" for "bus" and "coo" for "school")
- Sound substitutions ("wamb" for "lamb" and "tee" for "see")
- Sound distortions—the child attempts to make the correct sound but pronounces it incorrectly. (A distorted "s" sound may whistle, or the tongue may thrust between the teeth, causing a lisp.)
- Sound additions—extra sounds or syllables are added to a word ("animal" becomes "animamal")
- Speech may be unintelligible and hard to understand

How Is It Treated? Speech therapy for articulation problems involves helping the child to produce sounds correctly. Children with more severe articulation disorders are taught successive approximations—that is, the therapist will teach the child an approximate pronunciation of a word and work with her to get closer and closer to the correct pronunciation. (For example "toto" ⇒ "tayto" ⇒ "puhtayto" ⇒ "potato.") The therapist may use any number of different cues, such as verbal ("Put your tongue tip behind your front teeth."), visual (having the child look at the therapist's mouth or her own in a mirror), and tactile (having the child tap her mouth with her fingertip when making the "p" sound).

Auditory Processing Disorder

What Is It? Although their hearing is perfectly intact, children with Auditory Processing Disorder (APD) have great difficulty listening. And when you think about it, the act of listening isn't really a single act—children may have trouble with any number of aspects of listening: receiving, analyzing, organizing, storing, retrieving, and using information they hear. Because their brains aren't processing auditory information properly, children with APD struggle with understanding speech and developing language.

What Causes It? There isn't yet a clear answer as to what causes APD. Although it may coexist with other conditions, such as dyslexia, ADHD, and autism, it is not the result of these other disorders.

What Are the Signs?
  Some of these may be found in other conditions:
- Difficulty paying attention to information that's presented verbally
- Difficulty remembering information that's presented verbally; this is a problem with *auditory memory*
- Problems following multi-step directions
- May behave as if there is a hearing loss, often asking for repetition and clarification
- Struggles to pay attention to teacher because of inability to tune out background noises, also known as *auditory figure-ground* problems
- Difficulty identifying the origin of a sound, or *sound localization*

The most specific problems are as follows:
- Trouble distinguishing one sound from another (pat/pad, rice/rise); this is known as an *auditory discrimination* or *phonemic awareness* problem
- Difficulty identifying the similarities and differences in sound patterns (apple/appeal, apple/chapel), or *auditory pattern recognition*

How Is It Treated? The most successful treatment of APD involves three separate approaches: modification of the listening environment to reduce noise and enhance sound for the child, speech therapies designed to develop listening abilities such as decoding speech and improving auditory memory, and strategies that help the child compensate for the processing problem.

Dysarthria

What Is It? Dysarthria is a neurological speech disorder that limits the child's ability to use the muscles required for speech—lips, tongue, soft palate, larynx, and face—and, in turn, compromises his intelligibility of speech. Because of the child's oral-motor weakness, the result is often slurred or mumbled speech, as well as feeding and swallowing difficulties.

What Causes It? Weakened oral muscles may simply be present from birth or the result of any number of disorders involving the nervous system such as cerebral palsy, stroke, brain injury, or brain tumor. (In adults, dysarthria is often present in cases of Parkinson's, Lou Gehrig's, and Huntington's disease as well as multiple sclerosis.)

What Are the Signs?
- Slow, slurred, garbled, imprecise speech that is difficult to understand
- Inconsistent speech errors
- Articulation becomes less clear as the length of a phrase increases
- Inconsistent rate of speech because of poor motor control
- Limited tongue, lip, and jaw movement
- Inconsistent rhythm of speech
- Hoarseness or breathiness
- Drooling
- Chewing and swallowing difficulties

How Is It Treated? A speech-language pathologist will work with your child to slow his rate of speech, improve breath support so he can speak more loudly, and strengthen the oral muscles to improve his articulation. She'll teach you and your family strategies for enhancing communication. In severe cases, if your child is unable to speak intelligibly, an augmentative communication device may be considered and can take the form of something as basic as picture cards or as sophisticated as a computer.

Dysfluency/Stuttering

What Is It? Fluency is the natural flow of speech; when that flow is interrupted, it is known as dysfluency, or stuttering. Most children will experience some degree of dysfluency as part of the normal developmental process of learning language, usually between two and five years of age. The difference between these children and those with a true stuttering problem is the type and amount of dysfluency.

Developmental dysfluency usually appears in the form of repetition of whole words and phrases ("Let's go to go to the park.") rather than individual sounds and syllables ("Let's g-g-go to the p-p-park.") and tends to clear up as children mature and improve their communication skills. Children who stutter may do so in a variety of ways. There may be repetition of sounds (d-d-d-dog), syllables (mo-mo-mommy), parts of words (home-home-homework), whole words, and phrases. There may be stretching of sounds or syllables (vvvvideo), tense pauses between words, or speech that occurs in spurts. Often there are behaviors related to the stuttering, such as tense muscles (in the lips, jaw, and neck), tremors (of the lips, jaw, and tongue), foot tapping, eye blinking, and head turning. Your child may often speak quickly, become more dysfluent in stressful situations (talking on the phone is often challenging) than in talking with family and friends, and be easily frustrated. Because true stuttering can appear at the same age as developmental dysfluency—and because early treatment produces better outcomes—it's important to let a speech pathologist make that determination.

What Causes It? It is not entirely clear why children develop dysfluency, as there are many possible causes: genetic predisposition, poor coordination of the speech muscles, the way people talk to the child, and stress. According to an article from *American Family Physician*, stutterers have a neurophysical glitch that disrupts the precise timing required to produce speech. They may also have trouble coordinating the flow of air, articulation, and sound modulation.

What Are the Signs?
- Repetition of sounds (c-c-c-candy), syllables (da-da-daddy), parts of words (base-base-baseball), whole words, and phrases
- Prolongation, or stretching, of sounds or syllables (shooooes)

- Hesitations between words while the child is working very hard to get the sounds out
- Unusually long pauses before attempting to speak
- Five or more breaks per 100 words in the child's speech
- Heavy use of filler words such as "uh" or "um"
- Speech that occurs in spurts, as the child tries to initiate or maintain his voice
- Related behaviors such as tense muscles (lips, jaw, neck), tremors (lips, jaw, tongue), foot tapping, eye blinks, or head turns
- Variability in stuttering behavior depending on the situation, the person the child is talking with, and what the child is trying to accomplish
- A feeling of loss of control; child may feel embarrassed and may avoid troublesome sounds or words
- Avoidance of talking for fear of stuttering
- Abnormal breathing with speech

How Is It Treated? If your preschool child is experiencing dysfluency, or stuttering, there are two approaches a therapist may take: indirect and direct.

Indirect therapy is based on the idea that children's speech is influenced by their environment. The focus of treatment isn't on the child's stuttering, but rather on teaching the parents appropriate ways of interacting with their child so as to minimize any stuttering. Parents are instructed to speak at a slower rate, to wait a few seconds after their child speaks before responding (this slows the pace of the conversation), and to allow their child to finish speaking without interruption.

Direct therapy works on the premise that the dysfluency is the result of a speech-motor production problem. Treatment focuses on teaching your child to speak differently through modeling of easier speaking styles or through feedback about the child's fluency.

Therapy for school-age children, in addition to focusing on developing more fluent speech, also addresses the feelings, physical tension, and struggles associated with stuttering, as well as how to handle the reactions of others.

Expressive Language Disorder/Receptive Language Disorder

Also known as mixed expressive/receptive language disorder, specific language impairment.

What Is It? This particular disorder manifests itself in a variety of ways and, to add to the confusion, goes by a variety of different names. A child can have either expressive or receptive language difficulties; or she may have deficiencies in both areas and thereby be labeled "mixed expressive/receptive language disorder." While these terminologies are recognized by the medical profession through the *Diagnostic and Statistical Manual* (DSM-IV) and are used by practicing speech therapists, the research speech pathology community may refer to these same diagnoses as "specific language impairment" or, simply, "language impairment," often when describing children beyond preschool age who show no accompanying problems.

A child with expressive language disorder has difficulty choosing and combining words appropriately in order to communicate. She doesn't have trouble pronouncing words—that would be characteristic of an articulation or phonological disorder—rather, she has problems retrieving the right word, putting sentences together to communicate an idea, and using proper grammar. If she has trouble understanding spoken language, then she has a receptive language problem. Whether the deficit is receptive, expressive, or both, there is typically no obvious indication of a neurological, physical, sensorimotor, or social-emotional component.

What Causes It? Although the cause is not clear, there are a number of factors thought to play a role, such as your child's exposure to language and his skills in areas such as thinking and learning. Although the genetic origin hasn't yet been proved, studies show that 50–70 percent of children with expressive and/or receptive language disorder have at least one other family member with the disorder.

What Are the Signs?

Expressive

- Initial delays in babbling
- Slow acquisition of single words
- Delayed initiation of two-word phrases
- Word retrieval difficulties. She has trouble naming objects or "talks in circles" around a subject because she lacks the appropriate vocabulary.
- Misnames things or substitutes general words such as "thing" or "stuff"
- Difficulty grasping the rules of grammar
- Drops off "be" or "do" verbs when asking questions (*He like me?* instead of *Does he like me?*) beyond age four (and it's not part of the cultural dialect)
- Difficulty with prepositions (in, at, of), articles (a, the), plurals, and pronouns
- Difficulty with verb tense (*She ride the bike* instead of *She rides the bike*)
- Difficulty with the meaning of words or sentences
- Difficulty using language appropriately in conversation (may have trouble taking turns or staying on topic)
- No two-word combinations by twenty-four to twenty-six months
- Echoing words or phrases at three years
- Inability to retell stories or talk about past events at three to four years
- Difficulty with attention, memorization of facts, learning, or reading at six to seven years
- Child may sound younger than he is due to high number of language errors

Receptive

- Child doesn't seem to listen when spoken to
- Lack of interest in hearing storybooks read aloud
- Difficulty understanding complicated sentences
- Inability to follow verbal directions (may have no trouble following directions that are part of a routine, such as "put on shoes and grab your backpack")
- Difficulty understanding figurative language such as idioms and puns
- Gives inappropriate, off-target responses to "wh" questions (who, what, where)
- Repeats back words or phrases (echolalia)
- Repeats back a question before giving a response to it (re-auditorization)
- Language skills are below the expected age level and often below the levels of other developmental areas, such as thinking skills and problem solving

How Is It Treated? A speech pathologist can help your child to more fully develop an understanding of the underlying rules of language by modeling proper usage through hands-on activities, word drills, and by creating opportunities for your child to listen and respond. An individual program will be designed specifically for your child, based on which skills require attention.

Phonological Disorders

What Is It? Whereas an articulation disorder is the inability to physically produce sounds correctly, a phonological disorder is due to a child applying an incorrect rule of language. Children with this disorder are capable of making the appropriate sounds but fail to do so because they have not learned the rules of how sounds fit together, and may simplify words.

What Causes It? The cause of phonological disorder is not clear. Because a large proportion of children with this diagnosis have relatives with similar problems, it's possible there's a genetic component.

What Are the Signs?
- Errors are consistent
- Simplification of sound blends, also known as *cluster reduction* ("blue" becomes "boo" and "spoon" becomes "poon")
- Substitution of sounds produced in the front of the mouth (*t, d, n*) for sounds produced in the back of the throat (*k, g*), referred to as *velar fronting* ("gut" sounds like "dut," "car" becomes "tar," and "go" comes out as "do")
- Although a sound may be pronounced correctly in some words, the child may pronounce it incorrectly in others depending on where the sound falls in the word. (For example, he may be able to pronounce the "g" in "go" and the "b" in "ball," but may have trouble with the same sounds at the end of words, so "pig" becomes "pi" and "tub" is "tuh.")
- Children are frequently unintelligible and may only be understood by their parents

How Is It Treated? The speech therapist will work with your child to make him aware of the correct sound rules and will drill him with these patterns. One effective technique is referred to as *minimal pairs* and involves presenting the child with pairs of words and helping him to discriminate, and produce, the differences between sound patterns, such as "block/lock" and "nut/gut."

Semantic Pragmatic Language Disorder

What Is It? There is some debate over how exactly to categorize Semantic Pragmatic Language Disorder (SPD). Some experts believe it is purely a language disorder; others view it not as its own distinct diagnosis, but rather as a descriptive term to describe the communication difficulties of children with Asperger syndrome, autism, or nonverbal learning disability, a neuropsychological disorder associated with difficulty in reading nonverbal communication. However you and your child's doctor and SLP choose to identify this disorder, its characteristics remain the same. Semantics is the aspect of language related to understanding the meaning of words, phrases, and sentences, as well as using words appropriately when we speak, including abstract concepts and idioms. Pragmatics refers to how we use language in a social setting, such as knowing what is appropriate to say (as well as where and when to say it) and being able to participate in the give and take of conversation. It also includes understanding and using the appropriate tone of voice, intonation, and nonverbal behaviors necessary for successful social interaction. Children with Semantic Pragmatic Language Disorder struggle with the meaning of language in a social context. They have difficulty understanding the literal meaning of words and sentences, abstract concepts, words about emotions, idioms, and humor. They are unable to grasp the central idea of a story and may be disorganized in their own storytelling. They do not understand the rules of conversation, such as making eye contact, staying on topic, and taking turns.

What Causes It? Some believe SPD is the result of biological or neurological differences in the brain; it's also possible there's a genetic component. Children who have expressive language difficulties, or a diagnosis of autism, will have issues with semantics and pragmatics.

What Are the Signs?
- May appear inattentive or impulsive
- Difficulty listening and easily distracted
- Use phrases they've previously heard but may not understand
- Delayed speech; early vocabulary is mostly nouns
- Doesn't initiate pretend play

Parent to Parent

"Payton really had no idea what I was saying to him. Once his sister reached sixteen months, I could see the things he wasn't doing. His receptive skills were terrible. He could not mimic us. He was extremely good at memorizing things, and I am really predictable. We did the same things, the same way, so with me, I thought he was getting it . . . but with a stranger he would just stare at them blankly whenever they would talk to him."

—Kelly, mom to five-year-old Payton, receptive and expressive delay, semantic and pragmatic language issues (Milwaukee, Wisconsin)

- Only talks about specific areas of interest
- Difficulty initiating, joining, and taking turns in a conversation
- Excessive questioning
- May have trouble staying on topic
- May have difficulty expressing feelings
- Doesn't make eye contact or use facial expressions appropriately
- Unable to interpret body language and facial expressions
- Doesn't understand jokes, idioms, sarcasm, abstract concepts
- Difficulty understanding the point of view of another person

How Is It Treated? Therapy will likely include a social language or social skills class in order to give your child the opportunity to practice his conversational skills in a realistic, yet safe, group of his peers. The speech therapist serves as moderator for the group and teaches the children how to begin and maintain a conversation, how to solve problems, how to work as a team, and how to read body language, among other crucial social skills. In a one-on-one setting, the SLP may use *social stories*, a method in which appropriate social behaviors are presented in the form of a story, to help your child learn how to interpret and behave in different situations.

Voice Disorders

What Is It? If the quality of your child's voice doesn't seem right—it's hoarse or breathy or it doesn't seem to match your child's size, age, or gender—she may have a voice disorder. Voice disorders in children are most often caused by vocal abuse—excessive use of the voice when talking, singing, and yelling, as well as coughing and throat clearing—and they take many forms. The most common vocal disorders include:

- **Laryngitis:** an inflammation of the vocal cords, caused by excessive use of the voice, infection, inhaled irritants, or the backup of stomach acid into the throat (known as gastroesophageal reflux, or simply reflux).
- **Vocal nodules:** benign growths on the vocal cords, caused by vocal abuse or reflux.
- **Vocal polyps:** soft, benign growths similar to a blister, caused by an underactive thyroid (hypothyroidism), reflux, or chronic vocal abuse.
- **Vocal cord paralysis:** occurs when one or both vocal cords doesn't open or close properly and is caused by head trauma, neck injury, tumor, certain neurological disorders, or viral infection.

Less common disorders among children include:

- **Contact ulcers:** sores or tissue that has worn away on or near the voice box cartilages. This occurs through misuse of the voice when the vocal cords are excessively forced together. May also be caused by reflux.
- **Laryngeal papillomatosis:** a rare disease caused by the human papillomavirus (HPV) that results in the growth of tumors inside the voice box, vocal cords, or the air passage from the nose to the lungs.

What Causes It? In addition to the common causes of vocal abuse and reflux (as well as other examples cited above), voice disorders may also be brought on by environmental conditions such as allergies or cigarette smoke, chronic throat clearing, or dryness from medication. Children born with congenital abnormalities or who have had long-term intubation owing to premature birth or another medical condition may experience voice difficulties. Physical irregularities such as a cleft palate (a split in the roof of the mouth) or velopharyngeal insufficiency (the improper closing of the soft palate muscle during speech) can also cause vocal difficulties.

What Are the Signs?
- Chronic hoarseness, harshness, or breathiness, also known as *dysphonia*
- Voice is always too loud or too soft
- Pitch is inappropriate for the child's age or gender
- Frequent voice breaks, as though the child's voice cuts out for a second
- Frequent pitch breaks—fleeting, abrupt changes in the pitch of the child's voice
- Recurring temporary loss of voice, especially first thing in the morning or at the end of the day, referred to as *intermittent aphonia*
- Voice sounds strained as though speaking requires special effort

How Is It Treated? Depending on the exact nature of the voice disorder, treatment might include surgery (for vocal paralysis and laryngeal papillomatosis). Medication may be prescribed to treat allergies or reflux that are contributing to the problem. If it's determined that chronic throat clearing is characteristic of a tic disorder, medication or cognitive therapy may prove helpful. Keeping the child's home smoke-free is also important. Children must also develop an awareness of their vocal patterns in order to modify their behavior.

A speech pathologist will use tapes of appropriate and inappropriate vocal productions to help the child's understanding. Behavioral management programs that use positive reinforcement are effective in eliminating abusive vocal behaviors.

COEXISTING CONDITIONS

You might think that the speech and language issues we have discussed here are enough of a challenge. But, many children also experience additional conditions that, on the surface, seem to be distinct from their communication impairment. There exists a high rate of coexisting conditions with speech and language disorders. Some in the field think that when there is more than one disorder, both are actually symptoms of a broader underlying condition, even if that condition doesn't have a name yet.

Hypotonia

Muscle tone is the amount of tension or resistance to movement in a muscle. Children with low or decreased muscle tone are said to have hypotonia, and are characterized by problems with mobility and posture, breathing, feeding, and speech difficulties, ligament and joint laxity, and poor reflexes. While most children tend to flex their elbows and knees when resting, hypotonic children hang their arms and legs by their sides; this, along with their poor head control, gives them a "floppy" appearance.

Although hypotonia may be the result of genetic, muscle, or central nervous system disorders (such as Down syndrome), its cause is often unknown.

Children with hypotonia may have poor trunk support, that is, they have trouble holding their body upright. This poor body positioning can have an impact on their breath control, which in turn affects their speech. Low muscle tone can also affect the facial muscles and contribute to a child's rate of speech, quality of voice, and ability to move the tongue, lips, jaw, and palate. As a result, speech may be slowed, slurred, or nasal.

Physical therapy can improve motor control and overall body strength. Occupational and speech therapy can help breathing, speech, and swallowing difficulties as well as fine motor skills. While hypotonia can be a lifelong condition, in some cases, muscle tone can improve over time.

Sensory Integration Disorder

Sensory integration is the body's ability to process information received through the senses. Hear the dog yelping in the other room? That's your ears receiving the information that your daughter is pulling his tail. Did your toddler just announce there's something in his diaper? I don't have to tell you the kind of "information" your nose will process on that one.

Most of us don't realize that in addition to the core five senses—taste, smell, sight, sound, and touch—we are constantly receiving additional information through our nervous system. Structures within the inner ear detect movement and changes in the position of the head. Components of muscles, joints, and tendons provide awareness of body position. These two senses are known as the *vestibular* and *proprioceptive* systems, respectively.

Sensory integration disorder (also known as sensory integration dysfunction or dysfunction of sensory integration) is when there's a glitch that prevents the brain from analyzing, organizing, and integrating sensory messages. A child with sensory integration difficulties is unable to respond to these messages in a productive or consistent way. He may have trouble using this information to plan and organize what he needs to do.

If his brain registers sensations less intensely than normal, he may demonstrate sensory-seeking behaviors: purposely bumping into walls or people; excessive swinging, twirling, or rocking; speaking too loudly; seeming to be unfazed by unpleasant odors; and tasting inedible objects.

If his brain registers sensations too intensely, he may demonstrate sensory-avoidance behaviors: having strong negative reactions to getting dirty or to the feel of certain clothes; avoiding running, climbing, or swinging; complaining about loud noises such as blenders or vacuums; objecting to odors that other children do not notice; and refusing to eat certain textures of foods.

How does sensory integration impact speech and language development? Think of it this way: Imagine someone is giving you driving directions. You need to listen, process the information, and ask appropriate questions. But all you can think about is how the tag in the back of your shirt is making you itchy and the hum of the refrigerator is hurting your ears. (Your brain is interpreting these messages more intensely than it should.) You're starting to lose focus, so you start hitting yourself in the head. (The proprioceptive input helps your body organize the sensory information it is receiving.) Now . . . are you supposed to turn left or right at the gas station?

Sensory integration dysfunction "intensifies the bigger problems of children with . . . serious language difficulty," according to Carol Stock Kranowitz in her book *The Out-of-Sync Child: Recognizing and Coping with Sensory Integration Dysfunction*. These kids have trouble focusing, are easily distracted, and have difficulty interacting with others. Their ability to function in the world is impeded by their very own central nervous system. So you can see how developing speech and language skills—really, any skills—becomes quite challenging.

In addition, Kranowitz discusses the connection between the vestibular system, which moderates our sense of movement, and the auditory system. The sensations of movement and sound both begin to be processed in the receptors of the ear, so it's not surprising that the vestibular system plays a key role in developing auditory processing skills. Kranowitz says we acquire the skill of comprehension just as we integrate vestibular sensations and, over time, we learn to interpret what we hear. So the child who has trouble processing vestibular input may have poor auditory processing skills.

Lastly, think about all the muscles of the throat, tongue, lips, and jaw that are required for the physical production of speech. The vestibular system also helps maintain muscle tone and influences motor planning—both of which are necessary for intelligible speech—so you can see how a dysfunctional vestibular system can contribute to communication difficulties.

DISORDERS ASSOCIATED WITH SPEECH AND LANGUAGE DIFFICULTIES

Sometimes a child's communication difficulties are symptomatic of a broader diagnosis beyond that of speech or language. For example, some children who may appear to have an auditory processing problem may in fact have Attention Deficit/Hyperactivity Disorder (ADHD). Because these kids have trouble focusing during conversations and verbal directions, they give inappropriate responses and demonstrate poor memory skills. There's nothing wrong with their ability to process; rather, their impulsivity and distractibility contribute to communication difficulties.

So while the following diagnoses are not considered communication disorders, they are still characterized by speech and language difficulties.

Attention Deficit/Hyperactivity Disorder

Attention Deficit/Hyperactivity Disorder (ADHD) is a neurobiological disorder characterized by inattention, impulsivity, and hyperactivity. All children will at some time have difficulty with one or more of these areas. I've no doubt that most children, when asked to turn off the television so they can start their homework, appear inattentive, just as a three-year-old walking past the cookie aisle in the supermarket seems impulsive when he grabs a couple of boxes off the shelf. These are developmentally appropriate behaviors. But when they continue beyond a certain age, when the behaviors are so persistent that they interfere with the child's everyday functioning, it may be ADHD. Children with attention deficit issues have great difficulty controlling their behavior. As Martin L. Kutscher, M.D., writes in *ADHD Book: Living Right Now!* "People with ADHD cannot inhibit the present moment long enough to consider the future."

Children with ADHD may:

- Have difficulty listening and attending to conversations and classroom lessons
- Function similarly to children with auditory memory and processing difficulties. Kids with ADHD have poor auditory memory because they're likely not paying attention—not because they're unable to retain information. Likewise, there is nothing wrong with their processing systems; rather, they fail to attend to the appropriate information.
- Interrupt others or speak out of turn in class
- Struggle with the rules of social language (pragmatics) such as taking turns in conversation and staying on topic
- Have difficulty telling a story, from beginning to end, in a clear and efficient way

Autistic Spectrum Disorders

Autism is a developmental disability that typically appears during the first three years of life. It's the result of a neurological disorder that affects the normal functioning of the brain. Children on the autistic spectrum have difficulties with three key areas of development: social interaction, verbal and nonverbal communication, and imaginative play. As a spectrum disorder, autism takes several different forms and affects each child differently. According to the current classification system, autism actually falls under the broader category of pervasive developmental disorders, of which there are five distinct diagnoses: autistic disorder, Asperger syndrome, childhood disintegrative disorder, Rett disorder, and pervasive developmental disorder—not otherwise specified (PDD-NOS).

Children with autistic spectrum disorders may:

- Be delayed in the amount of language used or may be unable to speak at all
- Have difficulty understanding the meaning of words (semantics)
- Have trouble interpreting facial expressions
- Fail to understand verbal humor or idioms
- Have unusual intonation and may sound robotic, sing-songy, or whispery
- Repeat words and phrases they've heard before (echolalia)
- Use stock phrases to start a conversation
- Repeat the same word or phrase over and over (perseveration)
- Have a poor attention span
- Be unresponsive when others are speaking to them
- Have trouble with the rules of social language (pragmatics)
- Avoid eye contact and not respond to their name
- Have impressive vocabularies and be very articulate, but only about those topics that are of interest to them. They often "lecture" others rather than engage in conversation. (This applies only to kids with high functioning autism, such as Asperger syndrome.)

Cognitive and Intellectual Disabilities

Cognitive and intellectual disabilities are characterized by significant limitations in intellectual functioning and adaptive behavior. Intellectual functioning refers to one's ability to learn, think, solve problems, and make sense of the world and is measured by an IQ test. The average score is 100. Those who score below 70 to 75 on the IQ test, and have limitations in adaptive behaviors, can be described as having an intellectual disability previously referred to as mental retardation. Adaptive behaviors are those skills necessary to function in everyday life and include conceptual (receptive and expressive language, money concepts), social (responsibility, interpersonal), and practical (dressing, eating) skills.

Children with cognitive and intellectual impairment may:

- Take longer to learn to speak and have trouble speaking
- Be developmentally delayed in many areas
- Have trouble remembering things
- Lack an understanding of social rules

Down Syndrome

Down syndrome is a genetic disorder, the result of an extra chromosome that includes a combination of physical, intellectual, and developmental delays and difficulties. There is often some degree of cognitive impairment and characteristic physical features that include slanted eyes, small ears, flattened nose, short stature, and "floppy" appearance due to low muscle tone. Physical problems may include heart defects, problems with vision and hearing, and increased risk for infections, thyroid problems, and leukemia.

Children with Down syndrome may:

- Have a mild to moderate hearing loss
- Speak their first words between two and five years of age
- Have receptive skills that are more developed than their expressive skills
- Exhibit expressive language deficits, especially in syntax
- Have difficulty being understood by others
- Have auditory memory problems

- Have structural differences in the size and shape of their mouth that affect their clarity of speech
- Speak in a distinct, and often hoarse-sounding, voice
- Speak with a stutter

Hearing Impairment

Hearing loss in children is typically caused by one of three factors: otitis media (ear infection), congenital causes, and acquired causes. Recurrent ear infections can cause damage to the eardrum, the bones of the ear, and the hearing nerve, resulting in a permanent, sensorineural hearing loss. Congenital (at birth) hearing loss may be the result of genetic factors or any number of conditions such as maternal diabetes, infections, or complications associated with the Rh factor in the blood. Acquired hearing loss can occur anytime after birth, and common causes in children include infections, certain medications, meningitis, influenza, head injury, and noise exposure. There are three basic types of hearing loss:

- **Conductive:** Hearing loss occurs when sound is not conducted efficiently through the outer ear canal to the eardrum and the tiny bones of the middle ear. This type of hearing loss usually involves a reduction in the ability to hear faint sounds and can often be medically or surgically corrected.
- **Sensorineural:** Hearing loss occurs when there is damage to the cochlea (inner ear) or to the nerve pathways from the inner ear to the brain and cannot be corrected.
- **Mixed:** When there is damage in the outer or middle ear as well as the inner ear or auditory nerve, the hearing loss is considered a combination of conductive and sensorineural, or mixed.

Children with hearing loss are at a great risk of delay in both receptive and expressive communication skills. If not addressed early on, this can lead to learning problems, social isolation, and poor self-esteem. Research indicates that children who receive intervention early on may be able to develop language equal to that of their hearing peers.

Children with hearing impairment may:

- Have trouble hearing speech, especially quiet speech sounds such as *s, sh, f, t,* and *k* and therefore do not include them in their speech
- Have trouble hearing word endings such as –s or –ed. This leads to misunderstandings and misuse of verb tense, pluralization, nonagreement of subject and verb, and possessives
- Speak too loudly or too softly because they can't hear their own voice
- Have a vocabulary that develops more slowly
- Learn concrete words (cat, jump, red) more easily than abstract words (before, equal to, jealous)
- Have difficulty understanding words with multiple meanings
- Have difficulty understanding and writing complex sentences, such as those with relative clauses ("The teacher whom I have for math was sick today.") or passive voice ("The ball was thrown by Mary.")

SPECIAL CONSIDERATIONS

Parents raising children adopted from overseas, or in a home where more than one language is spoken, may find themselves experiencing communication challenges unique to both these situations. That doesn't mean all children in these environments will have difficulty, but it is something parents should keep in mind.

International Adoptions

Children initially raised in institutional settings often don't receive an appropriate level of language stimulation; they may miss vital precursors to language development such as eye contact, positive feedback, and the consistent back and forth communication that typically occurs between a parent and child. This lack of stimulation is compounded when the child comes from a country where income levels are low and both nutrition and health care services are below standard. In addition, when these children experience an abrupt change in language, they tend to stop using their first language while acquiring their new one.

The combination of inadequate stimulation and switching languages places internationally adopted children at risk of developing speech and language disorders. According to an article in the *American Journal of Speech-Language Pathology*, there is a lack of solid data on the prevalence of communication disorders among internationally adopted children. That said, the issue is one of concern to adoptive parents: researchers at the University of Wisconsin found that 57 percent of internationally adopted children were seen by speech-language pathologists.

As a first step, adoptive parents should have their child's hearing tested. A comprehensive physical examination of your child will determine if there are any physical reasons for a language delay. A speech pathologist will need to determine whether your child's communication difficulties are simply the result of a typically developing child who is still learning English or of a language-disordered child who struggles to learn any language. It is important that these children are evaluated in their native languages; if they are having trouble with their first language, they will certainly struggle to learn English without the proper intervention.

Bilingualism

Parents of bilingual children may have concerns about how their bilingualism may affect their language development. But there's no need. "There is no evidence that hearing more than one language ultimately slows speech and language development," says Brian Goldstein, Ph.D., acting chair, communication sciences at Temple University and editor of *Bilingual Language Development and Disorders in Spanish-English Speakers*. "Parents should speak in the language in which they are most comfortable."

When children are exposed to two languages from infancy on, they learn more quickly when each language has its own cues. For example, the mom may speak English and the dad may speak French. Or parents may have their children speak Spanish at home and English at school. It's not uncommon for some of these kids to combine the two languages to create a version of their own. But if there are concerns, a speech therapist would need to consider the child's vocabulary size in both languages.

For children who don't learn a second language until they are older, there are a series of stages that most second-language learners will experience.

Parents shouldn't be surprised if they notice their children going through a *silent period*—a common phenomenon during which children speak very little as they concentrate on listening to and understanding their new language. As they learn English, children may experience a *language loss*; they lose skills and become less fluent in their native language if it is not reinforced. This is called *subtractive bilingualism*. Ideally, children should experience *additive bilingualism*, where they learn English while their first language is maintained.

Children learning English as a second language may also *transfer rules* from their first language. For example, in Spanish, "esta casa es mas grande" means "this house is bigger." But a literal translation would be "this house is more bigger." A Spanish-speaking child producing this error would be demonstrating a language difference, not a disorder. Similarly, the Filipino child who says, "With my teacher, I have utang ng loob [debt of gratitude] because she has been so good to me," is demonstrating something called *code switching*, when a bilingual speaker changes languages within a given sentence.

Over time, bilingual children develop their speech and language skills as do their single-language-speaking peers. "If a bilingual child has a speech or language disorder, it should exist, albeit somewhat differently, in both languages," says Goldstein. Parents taking their child to a speech pathologist for an evaluation should expect their child to be assessed in both languages whenever possible. It is crucial that the SLP be able to distinguish between a child with a disability and one who is simply going through the normal process of acquiring a second language.

Hopefully you now have a better understanding of your child's particular speech and language issues. Don't be surprised if you see your child in more than one of the descriptions in this chapter; it is possible to have more than one diagnosis. Or your child may have only some of the characteristics of a particular disorder rather than the full description you read. You'll get a clearer idea after you talk with a speech therapist and have your child thoroughly evaluated. What's most important is that you get an accurate diagnosis and description that will guide the type of therapy your child gets. The next chapter delves into the different therapies used for each of the speech and language problems we've discussed here.

5

How They Do It: Understanding the Different Therapeutic Techniques

In the beginning, the Cookie Monster technique worked best for Max.

His therapist, Jenny, would prompt Max to imitate simple vowel sounds in exchange for little plastic chocolate chip cookies. Even an attempt from Max would net him another cookie. After he had all the cookies, Jenny turned on the battery-operated Cookie Monster toy—basically a figurine of Cookie Monster holding a cookie jar. Once it was activated, the jar lid automatically opened and closed and the furry blue guy turned around in circles. Max had to toss each cookie into the jar.

For Max, entering Jenny's room wasn't so much visiting someone's office as it was walking into an exceptionally well-stocked toy store. On any given day, the two of them might pretend to be dogs in a pet shop, pirates on a ship, or cars on a racetrack. Using her schnauzer, swashbuckler, and sports car, Jenny was able to pull sounds, words, and eventually, sentences from Max. Ari's therapist, Diane, also took advantage of her interests in order to get her excited about doing her work. And thanks to Ariel, Cinderella, Sleeping Beauty, and all their princess peers, "work" was always much more like "play" for Ari.

It is the job of all speech therapists to do two things: capture—and hold—your child's attention and interest, and provide engaging opportunities for your child to work on his specific issues while working toward a set of preestablished, long- and short-term goals. Much of therapy revolves around creating opportunities for your child to practice ideal speech and language, rather than repeat what is immature or inaccurate. *How* to do this will depend on many factors, including your child's diagnosis, age, temperament, interests, and of course, your child's speech pathologist. A three-year-old with expressive language disorder would not receive the same therapy as a seven-year-old with fluency problems. A child with severe apraxia might require intensive one-on-one therapy while a child with social language difficulties might benefit from a group therapy setting.

Just as the different speech and language diagnoses vary in nature, so, too, do the therapies used to treat them. Let's take a look at some of the strategies and techniques you may come across during your child's treatment.

NATURALISTIC VS. DIRECTIVE THERAPY

There are two overall approaches when it comes to how a therapist may work with your child: naturalistic and directive.

Naturalistic therapy—like Max's Cookie Monster game—blends the actual work of therapy with the natural, organic course of play. The child's opportunities for learning are spread throughout the session, as the therapist offers a variety of toys, games, puzzles, and art projects to work toward the child's goals. For example, if the therapist is trying to elicit bilabial sounds (speech sounds that require both lips for articulating, such as *b*, *p*, and *m*), she might set out a family of dolls that encourages your child to naturally label each one as *baby*, *mama*, and *papa*. With a naturalistic approach, the therapist plans the day's activities based on the child's individual interests and often follows the child's lead. It wasn't uncommon for Jenny to have several activities planned for Max, only to have him express interest in a game on her shelf. She'd allow Max to play his requested game while she still managed to incorporate the day's work into it. A naturalistic environment may not appear structured, but the therapist always has a plan for your child's goals and is flexible in meeting them in more creative ways.

Directive therapy is more structured than naturalistic, with the therapist directing the events of the session. She'll use larger blocks of time for drill work, for example, working on word approximations of increasing difficulty. She'll model the correct pronunciation of a word and then prompt your child to do the same. ("Pu-ppy. You say 'pu-ppy.' ")

Your child's therapist will take several things into consideration when choosing which approach to take: your child's personality and disposition, his age and stage of language development, and his conversational skills. For some kids, a directive-based therapy can be very effective in the beginning stages when the goal is to teach a new skill, such as speaking simple verbal responses. A more naturalistic approach may be used for encouraging the child to incorporate new skills into different settings, such as increasing spontaneous language and maintaining a conversation.

A good therapist will incorporate both approaches into her practice, depending on the needs of her clients. She may take a directive approach while still allowing the child to make some choices. ("Today we're going to work on *r* words. Do you want to play Don't Break the Ice or Hungry Hungry Hippos when we're done?") Or she'll use each approach as she sees fit. "I use a naturalistic approach with my preschoolers and a more direct approach with my upper grade students," says Mariann, a speech pathologist in Vienna, Virginia. "I rely on natural techniques for social language elements and direct ones for articulation, voice, fluency, and oral motor therapy. These are very specific areas that initially need to be addressed without the influence of other factors."

Professional Opinion

"A technique I use is 'my turn, your turn.' With those children who need the structure of directive therapy, I start out the session by asking, 'Do you want to start with play time or Darci time?' Darci time is up at the table. Play time is usually on the floor with the toys. If the child makes a choice, I give them the option. If not, I set a timer for five minutes and we play. When the timer goes off I say, 'Darci time' and we go sit at the table. Then I introduce the speech sound cards and play games with that. The timer rings again and I say, 'Oh, we have to stop working. It's play time.' And we get back on the floor and start the routine over again. What the kids don't know is that I am reviewing their mastered words and introducing new sounds and words during their play time. I have used this technique with children from twenty-four months to twelve years."

—*Darci Truax, speech-language pathologist (Gillette, Wyoming)*

ONE-ON-ONE VS. GROUP THERAPY

Speech therapy can be conducted on a one-to-one basis between child and therapist, or in a group setting with two or more children being instructed by one SLP. The decision on how to best service your child will be based on his age, developmental stage, the type and severity of his disorder, and, if applicable, any additional developmental challenges he may have.

One-on-one therapy can be especially important at the beginning stages of therapy so children can become familiar—and comfortable—with their therapist and learn what to expect from their ongoing sessions. Although an initial evaluation has already been conducted, these early days of therapy are important for the therapist to get a more complete look at your child in a nontesting environment and determine which goals should be addressed first.

One-on-one therapy is best for establishing new skills and teaching rules of language, such as proper articulation, appropriate pronoun usage, or any skill that could be taught through drills. It's also crucial for treating children with severe disorders who might not achieve the same results, or achieve them as quickly, if they received group therapy alone. A one-on-one approach affords children with the privacy of a supportive environment in which to practice skills that may be difficult for them.

Group therapy can be as small as two children or as large as a classroom setting. The size, participants, and structure of the group vary depending on the needs and abilities of the children and the intervention techniques being used. For children working on pragmatic, or social, language skills, a group therapy environment is ideal. And in school settings where caseloads tend to be large and a therapist's time tends to be stretched, groups for children of the same age working on common goals are often the therapy of choice.

Groups allow children the opportunity to carry over the skills they've learned in one-on-one therapy into a more natural setting among peers. "It's a way to see if old speech habits crop back up once structured drills aren't being used anymore," says Jennifer Hill, a speech pathologist in Sylvan Lake, Michigan.

THERAPY STRATEGIES

Each speech and language diagnosis requires specific therapeutic techniques designed to address the difficulties associated with each disorder. That said, there are many general strategies all speech therapists employ to stimulate your child's communication and refine his speech. Your child's SLP will give you specific exercises to practice with your child at home, but it's also important to understand the strategies being used in therapy so you can begin to incorporate them into your own communication with your child. That consistency is key to your child's progress.

Direct Modeling

Direct modeling is a technique often used in the early stages of therapy and it involves the therapist "modeling" or providing an example of a specific speech target or goal. For example, if your child says, "That's a *bid* bird," the SLP might respond with, "Yes, it is a *big* bird. It's really *big*. Is he *bigger* than *Big* Bird on 'Sesame Street'?" The idea is for your child to hear the correct pronunciation within the context of natural conversation.

Indirect Modeling

Indirect modeling involves the therapist demonstrating a specific speech behavior in order to familiarize your child with frequent and correct examples. If the child is practicing correct pronunciation of the letter *s*, the SLP may use an unusually high number of words that begin with the letter *s*. She might say, "Do you *see* what I have in this *sack*? I *see* a *sticker*. I *see* a *soldier*. I *see* a *submarine*."

Prompts or Cueing

A prompt, or cue, can either be a verbal or nonverbal cue designed to help your child perform a particular task (known as a target), whether it's to clearly articulate a particular sound or to explain the next part of a story.

The SLP may use a prompt to gain your child's attention and have him focus on the current task ("Look at my mouth." "Are you ready?") or to give him instructions related to the task ("Remember to lift your tongue tip at the beginning of each word." "Make sure your answer has three words in it.").

A nonverbal cue might be a gesture to indicate that your child needs to speak in a louder voice or a hand movement, such as quickly touching the lips with the index finger, to remind your child that the words he's saying have a "popping" sound.

Successive Approximation

Because some communication tasks are too complicated to be performed successfully, your child's therapist will break them down into more manageable tasks. If your child is struggling with multisyllabic words, the SLP will practice first with smaller pieces of the word. For example, in order to teach your child to say *table*, the therapist may first work with him to say *tayo*, then *taybo*, and finally, *table*.

Expanding

Expanding is when the therapist rephrases what your child said into a more mature or complete thought. For example, if your child and the SLP are role-playing with dolls, your child might say, "Daddy cookie," The therapist will build on these two words and respond with "Yes, daddy is eating a cookie."

Fading

Once your child has mastered a particular skill, the speech pathologist will start to eliminate, or fade, the modeling that was required earlier on. For example, in the beginning of therapy, the SLP might have modeled a complete sentence: "The boy is running." Once the child is able to produce the complete sentence, the therapist only models part of the sentence—"The boy is . . . "—and waits for the child to complete it. From there the therapist may only need to say "The boy . . . " in order to elicit a complete response.

Oral Motor Therapy

Oral motor therapy uses nonspeech oral exercises—such as blowing bubbles or drinking through a straw—for the purpose of stimulating speech development and improving speech production. Its effectiveness is widely debated in the speech pathology community.

Proponents of oral motor therapy say it improves speech by heightening awareness of the oral structure, warming up the speech musculature and improving voluntary control of oral movements. And for children with true oral motor difficulties—such as poor feeding and drooling—oral motor therapy is a legitimate and widely recognized form of treatment. However, the use of this therapy for treating *speech* problems is where the controversy lies.

Those who challenge this form of therapy say that while the same structures are used for both speech and nonspeech tasks (eating, sucking, breathing), they *function* differently for speech and nonspeech activities; differences exist in how the nervous system organizes movements necessary for speech and nonspeech activities.

Critics contend that the only evidence to support the use of oral motor therapy for speech problems is anecdotal and not scientifically based. Gregory L. Lof, associate professor and associate director of the graduate program in communication sciences and disorders at the MGH Institute of Health Professions described ten studies evaluating the effectiveness of nonspeech oral motor exercises at the 2006 American Speech-Language-Hearing Association convention. Of those ten, nine showed no benefits. The one study that did demonstrate benefits had methodological flaws that called in to question the validity of the results.

With so many speech therapists practicing oral motor therapy, and with multiple programs and oral motor toys and tools being marketed, it can be difficult for parents to assess what is real and what is hype. As with any treatment you're considering, consider your child's needs and do your own research. Talk with other parents and consult your pediatrician and speech therapist about whether your child would benefit from oral motor therapy.

COMPUTER-BASED THERAPIES

Your child's speech therapist may recommend a computer-based therapy as part of his treatment plan. There are many programs on the market and we'll discuss two of them here. These treatments are based on the concept of neuroplasticity—the brain's ability to create new neural pathways through experience. These programs create very specific experiences meant to gradually build pathways of use to language function. One of the methods was developed by neuroscientists based on their research on the topic. The other originated as a tool to help musicians improve their timing and rhythm. Ask your child's therapist to see if either of these programs—or any others—would be worth trying. Be sure to ask your therapist to direct you to studies to show if the method was helpful to other children like yours.

Fast ForWord

Fast ForWord is a computer software program created to help children with language impairments develop the necessary skills for listening, speaking, and reading. It's based on the theory that some children have an auditory processing impairment underlying their language difficulties. The games are designed to lengthen and intensify individual sounds in order to help children discriminate subtle sound differences, build phonological awareness, and, eventually, teach the brain to process signals that gradually become more like normal adult speech.

There's a big time commitment for parents electing to have their kids try this program; the children play the games for close to two hours each day for five days a week. Once your child has mastered the necessary skills for the first level of the game, the software automatically moves him along to the next level. Although much depends on the individual child and how much he adheres to the program, most will complete the program within four to eight weeks.

Paula Tallal, a professor of neuroscience at Rutgers University and cofounder of Scientific Learning Corporation, the company that developed Fast ForWord, conducted a study with children diagnosed with specific language impairment. Following four weeks of daily use of the Fast ForWord program, the children made language gains of eighteen to twenty-four months, as measured by standardized testing of language comprehension.

Parents should note that there are researchers who believe that because Fast ForWord has not been evaluated in a clinical trial format, the results fail to meet scientific standards of evidence for broad general use.

Needless to say, there is some debate in the speech pathology community over the effectiveness of Fast ForWord for children with language impairment. The debate is even more intense when it comes to children with other disorders. So as with any treatment you may consider for your child, it's best to talk it over with your pediatrician and speech therapist.

Interactive Metronome

Interactive Metronome is a brain-based therapy using neuromotor exercises to stimulate the brain to adapt or create new neural pathways—known as neuroplasticity—that compensate for injury or developmental delay. Current research indicates that this therapy may improve motor planning and sequencing—both of which play a big role in the acquisition of speech, language, and cognitive ability.

How does it work? The child wears headphones through which he hears a steady beat. He is outfitted with a special glove and he stands on a floor mat—both with sensors that measure how well his hand and foot movements are synchronizing with the beat he hears. A computer provides visual cues, along with the auditory ones, to let the child know if his attempt is early, late, or right in rhythm with the beat.

According to Stanley Greenspan, clinical professor of psychiatry at the George Washington University Medical School and director of research for the Scientific Advisory Board of the Interactive Metronome, because motor planning and sequencing are fundamental to abilities such as attention, motor skills, and sequencing information, Interactive Metronome "has the potential to favorably influence development in a number of areas."

A study in the *American Journal of Occupational Therapy* identified five areas of statistically significant improvements gained through Interactive Metronome, including attention and focus, motor control and coordination, language processing, reading and math fluency, and regulating impulsivity.

AUGMENTATIVE AND ALTERNATIVE COMMUNICATION

Augmentative and alternative communication (AAC) refers to a variety of ways, other than speech, that are used to communicate. It's something we all use on a regular basis, probably without realizing it; facial expressions, gestures, and writing are all ways in which we supplement our spoken words.

But for children with severe speech or language problems, there are special augmentative techniques and devices designed to help them communicate as effectively as possible. Some of these methods rely on:

- **American Sign Language (ASL).**
- **Hand gestures.** Such as Baby Signs®, improvised signs, and modified ASL.
- **Communication displays.** A series of logically arranged graphic symbols that the user touches to express himself. Can be as simple as picture cards or as intricate as a computerized system. PECS (Picture Exchange Communication System) is one such system, often used for children with autism.
- **Electronic devices.** Input into a keyboard, or other control, allows the device to speak for the child.

Making the decision to have your child use AAC can be difficult for some parents, as they may feel they are giving up on their child's

Parent to Parent

"For the first four months of therapy Decker was completely nonverbal and wouldn't really make many of his usual 'eh' sounds for his therapist. So we started with PECS [Picture Exchange Communication System], then moved to sign language, until finally at twenty-six months he started making some sounds to go with signs. His therapist was then able to move to more verbal exercises, gradually phasing out signing over the next few months."

— *Frith, mom to three-year-old Decker, moderate-severe expressive language delay (Pleasant Hill, California)*

ability to speak. But AAC is intended to supplement your child's speech—not replace it. In most cases, it is used as a temporary support, one that is abandoned once the child develops verbal communication. Your speech therapist can tell you if your child would benefit from AAC, and if so, which method is right for him. She can also either train you and your child to use a particular system, or refer you to a service provider who specializes in AAC.

WHAT WILL MY CHILD'S THERAPY LOOK LIKE?

Even though Max and Ari had the same diagnosis of apraxia, not everything about their therapy sessions were the same. Their therapists played to their individual interests in order to engage them in the "work" of therapy, which meant Jenny made good use of action heroes and race cars for Max, and Diane always pulled out the baby dolls and Disney princesses for Ari. And whereas Jenny and Diane took a play-based approach to therapy, Miss C., the early intervention therapist, relied on a directive approach.

How your child's therapist approaches his sessions will depend on his age, personality, and the nature and severity of his disorder. Here is a brief overview of some of the therapies commonly used for the disorders discussed in Chapter 4: apraxia, articulation, auditory processing, dysarthria, dysfluency, expressive/receptive language, phonological, semantic-pragmatic, and voice.

Therapeutic Intervention for Apraxia

Children with apraxia require frequent, one-on-one therapy sessions. They do not respond easily to traditional articulation techniques. Rather than teach your child to recognize different sounds by ear, therapists will use visual and tactile cues to help him establish the necessary motor patterns to produce speech. They will use a mirror to help children see how their lips, tongue, and jaw move when they try different sounds. To raise your child's sensory awareness of his mouth they will have your child concentrate on how sounds feel and where the tongue needs to be for different sounds. And they will focus on the melody and rhythm patterns of connected speech.

Because speech is a complex motor skill, the SLP will rely on drilling—intense repetitive practice—to improve your child's speech, rather than a therapy approach that relies on cognitive learning, that is, through explanations and modeling.

The goal of therapy is to increase the child's voluntary control over the movements necessary for accurate speech production and improve his intelligibility. This is done, initially, through imitation. Your child's therapist may ask him to copy simple sounds she makes; if he's unable, she'll start with hand movements, facial expressions, or mouth movements as a way for him to learn how to imitate. She may teach him word approximations, such as *gaga* for *doggie*. Once he's able to speak simple approximations, she'll work with him to increase the length of his utterances as well as the clarity as she helps to increase his vocabulary.

For kids with highly unintelligible speech, an alternative communication system may be suggested to provide them with a more immediate means of communication they can use while their verbal skills are being developed in therapy. It may be as simple as picture cards or as high-tech as a computerized system. For some children, this will be a temporary measure; for those with the most severe cases of apraxia, it may serve as the child's long-term mode of communication.

Therapeutic Intervention for Articulation Disorder

Frequent practice is key to successful articulation therapy, so sessions tend to consist of drill exercises to help your child correct his pronunciation. Because many articulation errors are developmental in nature—that is, children aren't expected to master certain sounds until a particular age—your SLP will choose which sounds to target based on your child's age. She'll have your child imitate her directly or she'll use picture cards or toys to elicit a response. Once he reaches a predetermined level of mastery—for example, when he can produce an initial *d* as in *doll* 80 percent of the time—she'll move on to a new target, such as the final *d* as in *wood*. The targets will get increasingly difficult as your child reaches each goal, and the therapist will work with him to produce these new sounds not only during the course of therapy but in spontaneous conversation as well.

Cues may be used to help your child learn where to place his tongue or position his lips and may be verbal ("press your lips together"), visual (child is instructed to look at the therapist's mouth or at his own mouth in the mirror), or tactile (child is directed to slide his finger down his arm when making the *s* sound).

If there is reduced muscle tone in his oral-facial area, she'll work on increasing strength—and thereby improve articulation—with nonspeech movements such as puckering lips, smiling, and blowing.

Therapeutic Intervention for Auditory Processing Disorder

The most successful treatment for Auditory Processing Disorder (APD) involves three separate approaches:

"I'm not sure of the specific therapy techniques involved but I will say that my child responded well to the incorporation of play into the therapy session. When Jordan worked with a therapist who was less 'playful,' it was difficult to get her to focus on the session. It also worked well when Jordan shared her session time with another child. Although I feared that sharing the time might 'water down' the therapy experience, having another participant seemed to enhance the 'play' aspect of the sessions."

—*Sharon, mom to four-and-a-half-year-old Jordan, articulation disorder (Farmington Hills, Michigan)*

Direct Treatment. A speech therapist will work with your child to improve her auditory discrimination, phonemic awareness, language-building skills, and auditory memory using a variety of methods, including specially designed computer games. The therapist will also work on developing her auditory cohesion skills (required for higher-level listening tasks), which will help her draw inferences from conversations, understand riddles, and perform verbal math problems.

Compensatory Strategies. Your child will learn strategies for problem-solving, memory, attention, and other cognitive skills in order to minimize the effects of the disorder. She'll also be taught to advocate for herself, for example, by asking her teacher to talk more slowly or repeat information if necessary. As the parent, you, as well as your child's teacher, will need to make some adjustments in how you communicate with your child: making eye contact with her before speaking, keeping instructions brief, rephrasing misunderstood information rather than simply repeating. Rephrasing might take the form of shorter sentences, more basic vocabulary, or a simple variation on the meaning. For example, if your child doesn't understand when you tell her, "Invite your brother to join us for lasagna and salad," try rephrasing your request: "Tell Sam it's dinner time."

Environmental Modifications. In the classroom, the teacher should seat your child close to her desk and provide her with printed materials to supplement any verbal instruction. Acoustics can be improved with carpeting and bulletin boards. If necessary, an FM system—also called an auditory trainer—can be used. The teacher wears a small microphone and your child wears a headset and receiver. This helps your child focus her attention on the teacher's voice while minimizing background noise.

Therapeutic Intervention for Dysarthria

Dysarthria affects five distinct areas and treatment should address all of them. The goal of therapy for children with dysarthria is to improve their intelligibility and their speech motor control by:

- Establishing consistent, controlled exhalation of air to support speech production (respiration or breathing)
- Achieving efficient vocal fold closure during speech (phonation or making of sound)
- Decreasing airflow through the nose (hypernasality) by improving child's ability to generate air pressure in the mouth (resonance or voice quality)
- Improving speech production within the limitations of the underlying neuromuscular impairment (articulation)
- Increasing child's overall intelligibility (rhythm of speech)

The SLP will work with your child to reduce her rate of speech and may utilize a metronome, pacing board, or graduated stick. With the metronome, children are taught to pronounce one syllable per "tick." The pacing board is divided into sections and the graduated stick has bumps on it. The child must either tap one section of the board, or touch a bump on the stick, every time she pronounces a syllable. Since she can't move her fingers as quickly as her mouth, these tools help to slow her rate of speech and improve her intelligibility. The therapist will instruct her to emphasize all syllables in order to reduce distortion of vowel sounds as well as to exaggerate consonant sounds as a way of compensating for the dysarthria.

Other techniques include biofeedback, which involves electronic monitoring devices that help the child gain some voluntary control over previously unconscious body functions, such as respiration and extraneous oral movements, and delayed auditory feedback, in which the child's words are returned to her through headphones after an imposed electronic delay of a few milliseconds.

Some children may require prosthetic devices to replace the function of a missing or impaired speech component, for example, a mechanical lift to correctly position the palate. Surgery may also be an option.

For children with severe dysarthria, learning an alternative means of communication may be the best option; methods include sign language, alphabet boards, and picture systems, as well as computerized devices and speech synthesizers.

Therapeutic Intervention for Dysfluency

There are several methods a speech therapist may use with your child to decrease her rate of speech:

- Timed syllabic speech—The stutterer is taught to speak syllable by syllable, with each syllable stressed evenly
- Shadow method—Your child repeats the words spoken by the therapist
- Fluency initiating gestures—She'll learn gestures that help prevent dysfluent speech

- Altered auditory feedback (AAF)—When people who stutter speak or sing in unison with others, their dysfluency is often reduced. This is known as the "choral effect." Altered auditory feedback (AAF) devices re-create that choral effect by changing the way your child hears her voice, either by delaying it (delayed auditory feedback, or DAF) or by altering the frequency (frequency altered feedback, or FAF)

Strategies for speaking more fluently involve changes to the timing and physical tension involved in producing speech. One such strategy is *easy onset*, in which the child is instructed to exhale slightly before speaking and to gradually reach an appropriate volume level for conversation.

Your child will also learn how to reduce physical tension during moments of dysfluency. No technique for increasing fluency is 100 percent successful all the time. Reducing tension allows children to stutter more easily so they are able to communicate with fewer disruptions. The speech pathologist may teach your child *pull-outs*: when he experiences a moment of dysfluency, he is encouraged to stop in the middle of that moment, mentally rehearse the intended word, and then try again.

The therapist will also work on helping your child accept his dysfluency. By accepting their dysfluency, children stop struggling, they relax their muscles and are more likely to experience improved fluency. This acceptance of stuttering can actually lead to less stuttering and more effective communication.

Therapeutic Intervention for Expressive/Receptive Language Disorder

If your child needs help with expressive language, his SLP will start by selecting target vocabulary words for him to work on. Typically these are words relevant to your child's daily activities (*mom, shoes, school*), words that are important to him (*trucks, French fries, Spider-*

man), as well as action words (*eat, play, draw, sleep*). She may encourage him to label what he sees by presenting him with a container filled with small items and toys and asking him to name each one as it is removed. To work on action words, she may set up an activity such as making popcorn and label each action (*open* the box, *take* out the popper, *pour* the kernels, *close* the top). Once his vocabulary increases, she'll work on categories ("What animals are on a farm?"), opposites (big and _____), descriptions ("What does your mom's car look like?"), grammar (use of small words such as *on, in, under,* and *over*; plural forms, pronouns), and narrative skills ("Tell me what happened in *Little Red Riding Hood.*").

For receptive language difficulties, therapy consists of the therapist repeatedly presenting a target word as well as using an exaggerated intonation. If she's trying to teach the word *throw*, she may give your child a ball and ask, "Can you THROW the ball to me? Put your hands over your head and THROW it to me. That's right, THROW it over here. Great, you did it."

Therapeutic Intervention for Phonological Disorder

Children with phonological disorder have difficulty understanding the underlying rules of phonology, or how sounds are made. Their speech errors are due to implementing incorrect language principles—called *phonological processes*—which are strategies used by typically developing children to simplify the production of speech sounds. Therapy focuses on reducing a child's reliance on them.

For example, if your child is deleting final consonants (he says *ca* for *cat*), the SLP will engage him in an activity where using the final consonant will earn him a sticker or other small reward. Word pairs, such as bow/boat, toe/toad, and tea/team would be incorporated into a game with pictures of each item, and your child would need to say the words with the proper ending sounds in order to win. In the early stages of therapy, the SLP should offer praise for any response that demonstrates an understanding of the phonological process being taught; if your child typically says *ru* for *run* but says *rug* or *rut*, he'll get positive reinforcement for simply adding a final consonant, even if it's not the right one.

Therapy will also revolve around *distinctive features*—the ways phonemes are broken down into smaller categories based on how they sound. For example, understanding that a *b* sound makes a buzzing noise in your throat (also referred to as a *voiced* sound) and a *p* sound does not (*voiceless*) can be very helpful for the child struggling to understand the differences between sounds. He'll learn about other ways sounds differ from each other, for example, those that involve the lips (*labial*), such as *p*, *b*, *f*, and *m* and those that do not (*nonlabial*), such as *d*, *k*, *o*, and *s*.

Therapeutic Treatment for Semantic Pragmatic Language Disorder

Your child's speech therapist will take advantage of real-life situations to teach vocabulary, concepts, and behavior in different situations. She may role-play different scenarios ("What do you do at a birthday party?" "How do you order dinner in a restaurant?" "How do you greet your teacher?") or use games, videos, and books to help convey appropriate and inappropriate language and behavior. She'll work on establishing reciprocal conversations, becoming a more efficient communicator by telling a story in an organized way, and understanding the meaning behind verbal and nonverbal communications.

She may use social stories, a therapeutic technique originally designed to help autistic children understand social situations, to teach your child how to follow routines, do an activity, ask for help, or respond appropriately when feeling angry.

Some skills are best taught in a group situation, which is why many speech therapists offer social language classes. Children are typically grouped according to age, although individual diagnoses can vary. (Children with receptive/expressive language disorder,

Professional Opinion

"Children with language learning disorders don't catch the underlying humor of multiple meaning words. They are very concrete in their thinking. To help them become better communicators the resource room teacher and I would choose a popular Disney movie and have them watch it. So after they saw *The Lion King*, for example, we did science, language, and art projects relating to the savannah. Then I went through the movie and wrote out every idiom—such as monkey's uncle—and we taught the vocabulary as well as the double meanings of words. After about six weeks, when all the projects were completed, we had a party with food relating to the theme and we watched the movie again. This time, the kids laughed on their own at the humor that had bypassed them the first time."

—*Darci Truax, speech-language pathologist (Gillette, Wyoming)*

autistic spectrum disorders, Asperger syndrome, ADHD, and OCD may also need help with their social language skills.) With the speech pathologist running the session—and the children serving as each other's therapy partners—they learn how to start and maintain a conversation, stay on topic, make eye contact, read facial expressions, and understand others' point of view.

Therapeutic Treatment for Voice Disorders

The goal of treatment is to help children speak with a voice that is an appropriate pitch, volume, and quality for their age and gender. Depending on the cause of your child's voice disorder, treatment may include medication, surgery, or speech therapy, and as such, your SLP will work in conjunction with your child's doctor to determine the best course of action.

If your child's vocal irritation is the result of reflux (the backflow of stomach acids to the throat and voice box) or postnasal drip from allergies, medication may be prescribed to alleviate the symptoms and thereby improve voice quality.

Surgery may be necessary to remove cysts in the vocal fold, to treat paralysis of the vocal folds, or to repair congenital problems such as a laryngeal web, which is a web of tissue between the vocal folds that didn't separate on its own.

Speech therapy will focus on increasing your child's awareness of his vocal behaviors to eliminate forceful voicing, reduce loudness and muscle tension, and adjust his pitch. He'll learn how to improve his respiratory control as this, too, affects voice production. His SLP will discuss the importance of vocal rest—limiting how much talking he does—as a way to rest the vocal folds.

It's a lot of information to digest, I know. But once you start observing your child with his speech therapist, you'll get an even better understanding of the techniques and strategies being used. Chapter 9 will discuss what you can do at home to support the work being done in therapy. But next we'll look at what you need to consider when choosing the right therapist for your child.

6

Getting the Right Help: Finding and Evaluating Your Child's Speech Therapist

It's our first day with our new therapist, and I'm sitting in the corner of the room watching Max watch Jenny.

He is enraptured by her, staring intently at her face as she slowly and deliberately moves her mouth, pronouncing each word with care. I see Max's mouth move, barely, along with her, as if he's trying to say the words but nothing comes out. That's OK. The fact that he has attempted to imitate Jenny is milestone enough.

Max is having a hard time staying in his seat, but Jenny continues working with him as he stands at the table. She's flexible, allowing Max to take the lead but always managing to bring him back around to the task at hand. She has quickly hooked him with her action figures, wind-up toys, and a collection of animals large enough to fill five miniature zoos. She is using Kaufman cards—a set of flash cards designed by speech pathologist and apraxia expert Nancy Kaufman to help children develop word approximations—to elicit simple sounds from him, and when I hear Max say "ah" tears well up in my eyes. It's only day one but I know in my heart that I have found the person who will give my son the gift of speech.

Finding Jenny was a blessing. I can't say the same about all the therapists my children have worked with.

Miss C. was Ari's early intervention speech therapist, and I vividly remember the day I questioned if no therapy would be preferable to bad therapy. She and Ari were getting ready to color a snowman. She holds out the yellow crayon and the red one and asks Ari, "Lello?" Ari reaches for the yellow crayon but doesn't say anything. Then, in what can only be considered an act of cruelty, Miss C. pulls the crayon away from Ari and says, "It's OK if it's too hard for you to say." And she puts the crayons away.

You have to understand that children with apraxia can't perform on command. They may be able to produce some sounds and words on their own but are typically unable to imitate someone else—especially when there's an expectation. You would no sooner offer a child with apraxia a toy in exchange for a verbal attempt than you would promise a child who relies on a wheelchair a prize for taking a step; it's not that these kids don't want to do it—they *can't*.

Had Ari been my first child with apraxia, I most likely wouldn't have understood any of this right off the bat. But by the time she had joined the speech therapy club, I had already been a member for a year and a half. And I had spent five months watching Max work, unsuccessfully, with a therapist who also expected a word in exchange for something. As I watched his first SLP hold a ball out for Max—and withdraw it when he was unable to give her even a "ba"—I had no idea how unfairly my son was being treated. Now, as I watch Ari fail to acquire a crayon, there's a knot in my stomach. Because this time, I know.

I have a hard time bringing Ari back to Miss C. each week when I feel she's using completely inappropriate techniques with her. We're already paying the private therapist for two sessions a week, but Ari's best chance at making serious progress is with at least three sessions a week. Our insurance company has a limit on the number of visits it will cover, so we're counting on the free school services to supplement what Ari needs. I keep bringing her back, despite Ari's frustration and the gnawing feeling that this is all wrong, in the hope that frequency of service will trump technique and something positive will, in fact, come from this therapist's work.

I know how stressful it is to be told your child has a problem. More than anything, you want a solution. So you start surfing online, making phone calls, and setting up appointments in the hope of alleviating the burning need to get your child started in therapy NOW. I know what it feels like when you hear the clock ticking—I was four states away from home when we got Max's official diagnosis, and if I could have willed that plane home any faster I would have.

The thing to remember is that it's important to take the time to find not just *a* speech therapist—but the *right* therapist—for your child. It's OK to shop around to find the best match—someone with the right experience who clicks with your child. If you don't find him or her on the first try, you can always switch after your child has started treatment. Really, you can. Look, you wouldn't go back to a hair stylist who ignored your directions. You'd likely change doctors if yours was always rude. And if you were looking to hire a reading tutor/interior decorator/accountant you would ask for recommendations and shop around. The same rules apply here.

SO, TELL ME ABOUT YOURSELF

Of course you're going to have questions about your child's diagnosis, prognosis, and how to best help him. But first, ask the following questions about your prospective therapist.

What Is Your Educational Background?

A speech-language pathologist should have at least a master's degree. While a bachelor's degree provides an introduction to the theory of communication disorders and treatments, a master's level goes much more in-depth, giving the student a thorough knowledge of the theory of specific disorders. It is at the master's level that students receive practicum experience working with actual clients under the supervision of licensed SLPs.

Are You Certified?

In the United States, practicing SLPs are certified by the American Speech-Language-Hearing Association (ASHA), as indicated by the "CCC" (Certificate of Clinical Competence) after their name. This certification ensures that the SLP has met a minimum level of education and training in communication disorders, has agreed to follow ASHA's code of ethics—including issues such as professional conduct, provision of services, and record keeping—and has committed herself to continued professional development.

How Many Years of Experience Do You Have? Do You Specialize?

In most cases, the more experience the therapist has, the better a clinician she is. (Bear in mind that there are those therapists who become set in their ways, may not keep up to date on the latest research, or who fail to bring the necessary passion and energy to each therapy session.) But it's important to find someone who

Parent to Parent

"I believe that some newer therapists may actually work out better than their seasoned colleagues because they come with an energy and freshness that may make up for their lack of years of experience."
—*Sharon, mom to four-and-a-half-year-old Jordan, articulation disorder (Farmington Hills, Michigan)*

specializes in working with children, as not all SLPs are trained in pediatrics. Look for someone who has experience working with kids in your child's age group and with your child's diagnosis.

How Many Children Have You Worked with Who Have My Child's Diagnosis?

Speech therapists should have worked with at least several children with your child's diagnosis, preferably more.

Do You Have Parents Attend or Observe the Therapy Sessions?

Therapy is most effective when the therapist and the parents work together as a team. Ideally, you should be present in the room—at least in the beginning—so you can not only observe, but ask questions about what the SLP is doing. You'll want to adopt her techniques and strategies in order to facilitate communication with your child. After a while, you may want to move to the observation room and watch your child's sessions through a one-way mirror. You may need to do this right from the start if your child is distracted by your presence in the room. If the SLP isn't comfortable being observed, you shouldn't feel comfortable going with this SLP.

Unfortunately, because many school-based speech services aren't equipped with observation rooms, you may not be able to watch your child's sessions. You can ask to sit in on the session but don't be surprised if you're told no; many therapists feel children don't perform as well with a parent in the room. While this may be true, it is still important for you to know what's going on in therapy. Try sitting outside the therapy room with the door ajar so you can at least listen in. If this isn't possible, then insist on regular updates. You can always ask the SLP to keep a notebook detailing each session's goals, activities, and your child's performance. Even if you are able to observe, the notebook will help you remember what exercises or activities to use at home and how to do them. It will also serve as a record of your child's progress.

Do You Provide Parent Training or Activities for Working with My Child at Home?

It is essential that skills being taught in therapy are reinforced at home. If you leave all the work to the therapist, it's like putting a Band-Aid on a broken arm—not too effective. The SLP should not only supply you with "homework," but also instruct you in how to do the work with your child. If he's not giving you activities to do at home, ask for them. Insist on being provided with as much information as you want about your child's diagnosis and treatment. Your therapist should be able to provide you with basic information on speech and language development, your child's specific diagnosis, and any specific treatment methods he may be using. If he resists sharing information or seems to take offense, he's not the SLP for you. No one knows your child as well as you do. You want a therapist who accepts you and values your input as a member of your child's speech team.

Will I Get Regular Written Reports?

You should expect detailed written reports for your child's initial evaluation and any reevaluations that may be conducted down the road.

Of course you'll be given verbal ongoing updates of your child's progress—written ones in your child's speech notebook if his services are taking place during the school day—but you may want to request written reports as well. There's a lot of information to absorb, most of which will probably be new to you and technical in nature, so it's helpful to have a written report you can refer back to, as well as share with any other professionals you might consult about your child.

These periodic progress reports should let you know how much closer your child is to reaching his goals. Ask the SLP how often you can expect a progress report and if there's any charge for them. (Because of the time needed to write a detailed report, private SLPs may bill for the time, although usually at a lower rate than for therapy.)

Do You Work from an Office or Do You Come to My Home?

For one-on-one therapy, the therapist may either work from an office or come to your home to work with your child. Be sure to ask how your prospective SLP works and consider what would be best for your child. Is the therapist's office close enough to your home that the one, two, or three times a week you need to go there doesn't leave you feeling as though you're living in your car? Would your child be more comfortable working from home—or would the phone, the dog, and your two other children be too much of a distraction?

How Much Do You Charge? Do You Take Insurance?

The cost of private therapy varies depending on the expertise and location of the therapist as well as the particular needs of your child. Don't be shy in asking how much you can expect to pay. Will you need to pay your therapist after each session or can she bill you each month? Does she accept your insurance or will you have to pay the total cost upfront and submit your expenses for reimbursement? If she does accept insurance, can she help you get coverage for your child's therapy? Is she willing to write a letter on behalf of your child to appeal any rejected claims?

HOW'S IT GOING SO FAR?

Once you've gotten answers to your questions and you've found someone with the appropriate qualifications, give her some time to work with your child and get to know him. Those kids who are shy or have a hard time separating from a parent may need more time than others to get comfortable with their SLP. Some kids, motivated by a room filled with games, toys, dolls, and more, dive right in.

Either way, after you've had a chance to observe your child's therapist in action, ask yourself the following questions.

Does He Like My Kid?

Does he greet you and your child warmly and enthusiastically? Is he able to get your child to do the work and meet his goals while remaining flexible and creative in the choice of activity? Will he follow his lead? Does he "get" him?

"It's important to look for someone who is in charge of the session without *having* to be in charge," says Kelly, mom to five-year-old Payton. "The SLP should know when to back off and try something else."

If your child receives speech therapy at school, it may be harder to assess his relationship with the therapist. You can certainly try to observe a few sessions. But most schools aren't equipped with observation rooms, so you'll need the therapist's OK to attend since you'll be sitting in the same room with him and your child. You may or may not get an accurate read this way. Another way to determine how the therapist feels about your child is to ask yourself the next question.

Does My Child Like Her?

"Decker knows that once a week we get to 'play' with Pamela, and he visibly brightens when he is told its time to climb into the car to visit her," says mom Frith.

Professional Opinion

"An effective SLP is:

- Flexible and changes for the needs of the child
- Constantly learning and researching new ways to reach the child
- One who attends conferences
- Not the same therapist he or she was five years ago
- Able to say 'I don't know' "

—*Darci Truax, speech-language pathologist (Gillette, Wyoming)*

Your child's therapy is more likely to be successful if he is a happy, willing participant. Yes, speech therapy is work—but a good SLP will make the work feel more like play, and ideally you'll work with someone your child looks forward to seeing. If he refuses to get out of the car, perhaps it's time to look for someone else.

Is She Setting Clear, Reasonable Goals for My Child? Is She Using Appropriate Techniques?

Ask yourself: How do I feel when I observe my child in session? Am I seeing him being challenged—or overwhelmed and frustrated? Is he able to do the work being asked of him? Are you noticing improvements over time?

Does He Keep Me Updated with Feedback and Suggestions After Each Session?

Yes, your child's therapist may have back-to-back appointments; but she should still allow a few minutes after each session to discuss the work your child is doing and offer suggestions for you to try at home. "It's important that parents are given activity suggestions to do at home between therapy sessions," says Leslie Zimcosky, a Painesville,

Parent to Parent

"We have been with the same practice for six years. Maya has seen two different therapists during that time and I love them both. They don't try to B.S. me. They're able to explain the process and Maya's progress. For me, the most important part of the parent-therapist relationship is being able to talk with the therapist and ask questions and really understand where my child is in her work. They have really embraced my daughter and she feels safe with them."

—Rachel, mom to seven-year-old Maya, expressive/receptive language disorder (Dobbs Ferry, New York)

Ohio–based speech language pathologist. "This helps with carryover of goals and strategies into the child's natural environment."

Am I Being Treated as Part of the Team? Does She Take Me Seriously When I Express Concerns or Offer Ideas?

I knew Diane was the right therapist for Ari when within ten seconds of meeting her she said, "I've talked with Ari's previous therapist, but I want to know what you think because the moms always know what's going on." Although she is the one with the professional training, she acknowledged that the parents bring their own expertise to the table. You want an SLP who treats you as an equal member of the team, not one who talks down to you and dismisses your questions.

Is He Willing to Get Involved in My Child's School and Talk with the Teacher and School SLP?

Your SLP's participation in your child's therapy shouldn't end at his door. He should be willing to talk with your child's teacher and offer advice as to the best way to communicate with your child. If your child sees two therapists—private and school-based—they should both be willing to communicate to make sure they're on the same page. They don't have to have identical goals for your child, but their plans and approaches should work together. And your desire for them to communicate is reasonable and appropriate. He should be willing to write the school a letter advocating for your child's needs, or better yet, accompany you to any important meetings regarding your child's school services. (Bear in mind he may need to charge you for his time and these expenses may not be covered by your insurance.)

Is She Willing to Help Me as Well as My Child?

Parenting a child with speech or language difficulties is a challenge. And the child's disability impacts far more than just her ability to communicate. So a good SLP should do more than just help your child speak—she should be able to equip you with the tools you need to best help your child, whether it's homework exercises, the title of an inspiring book, or the name of a good psychologist who can help you and your family through this difficult time. She should be willing to write a letter to your insurance company to help you get coverage for services. She should be able to offer you resources as well as emotional support. A good SLP isn't put off when you burst into tears in her office.

As parents, we're ultimately the "expert" on our kids. So it's up to us to spend the time—and energy—finding the therapist who will work best with them. I hope this chapter helps to simplify your search.

In addition to traditional speech and language therapy, there are many alternative and complementary therapies that may be helpful to your child, several of which are covered in the next chapter.

7

Eating Fish, Riding Horses, and Other Help from Unexpected Sources: Will Your Child Benefit from Complementary Therapies?

I didn't completely understand how it would work, but that didn't stop me from spending eighteen dollars on a bottle of fish oil capsules in the hopes of improving Max's speech.

I don't recall how I first learned of the health benefits of fish oil, or essential fatty acids—probably from my many hours of surfing the Internet—but I knew enough: parents were reporting increases in their kids' verbal expressions, and if it didn't help Max, it certainly wasn't going to hurt him.

Well, I can't say the fish oil was a success—not because it didn't work, but because I couldn't get Max to take the pills. At three years old, he was just too small, sensory-defensive—and stubborn—to swallow the capsule. So I would prick it with a pin and try to disguise the contents in juice. Because of the strong fish odor, he refused it. And who could blame him? (Would you enjoy your orange juice with a mackerel chaser?) But because I was starting to see improvements in his speech as a result of his intensive therapy, I didn't pursue it.

It would be years later when I would turn to fish oil again, this time, to improve Max's ability to focus and even out his explosive moods. He was older—six years—and the pills were smaller, and this time I had great success. Over time, we found that the fish oil did an equally good, if not better, job of managing Max's behavioral issues than the prescription medication we had tried.

Our family wasn't alone in our experimentation with alternative and complementary therapies. According to the American Academy of Pediatrics, as soon as Max swallowed that first golden pill he joined the more than 50 percent of children with chronic or recurrent conditions who use what is now referred to as complementary, alternative, or integrative medicine.

WHAT IS COMPLEMENTARY AND ALTERNATIVE MEDICINE?

Complementary and alternative medicine (CAM) is a group of diverse medical and health-care systems, practices, therapies, and products that are not presently considered to be part of conventional medicine. (Think acupuncture, chiropractic, and dietary supplements.) Complementary medicine refers to those treatments used in conjunction with conventional medicine; alternative medicine is used in place of conventional medicine. Integrative medicine combines mainstream medical therapies and CAM therapies for which there is some high-quality scientific evidence of safety and effectiveness.

Sometimes there is scientific research to support these complementary methods. Sometimes there isn't. But there is plenty of anecdotal evidence—just ask any of the parents sitting next to you in that waiting room. Or go online to visit one of the countless websites, Listservs, and message boards to read what other parents have tried with their kids. Of course it goes without saying that not all children will respond to these techniques in the same way. Some may have minor success, others will see significant improvement, and some none at all. Some children may experience negative side effects, in which case you shouldn't hesitate to terminate that particular therapy.

There's no way to know which method will best serve your child. So, just as it's up to you to get your child a correct diagnosis and find the speech therapist who works best with him, you'll also need to investigate the various complementary and alternative treatments available for speech- and language-impaired children to see if any make sense for your child.

Assessing Alternative Treatments

The number of companies, health-care practitioners, and websites offering alternative therapies grows every day. Some may have merit; others may not. How are parents supposed to sift through all the information and make an informed decision regarding their child's treatment?

When considering therapy options and alternative treatments, ask yourself:

- **What is the source of the information?** You can trust what you read on the website of a government agency (such as the National Institutes of Health), nonprofit organization, national disorder-specific organization (such as ASHA), or medical school. But if it's a website that sells the products or services it touts in its online "articles," consider it a less objective source.
- **Is the research behind it valid?** There are two ways to evaluate treatments. The *standard scientific procedure* involves testing the treatment in controlled conditions, with enough subjects to give weight to the results. Good scientific studies go through a peer review before they are published in a scientific journal; another group of professionals reviews the research in order to confirm, or refute, the findings, or to at least ensure that the methods were appropriate and objective.

    In *limited case studies* or *testimonials*, conclusions are drawn from a limited sample size and are often based solely on testimonials from doctors or patients. This doesn't mean the treatment is harmful or ineffective—but without a standard scientific evaluation, it does raise questions about its effectiveness and safety.

- **Are the research findings preliminary or confirmed?** Often the media reports a preliminary finding as "breakthrough" when really more time, subjects, or research is needed for confirmation. Try to locate the original source, such as a professional scientific publication, to get a better understanding of the reported findings.

- **Is the information believable?** Approach with caution any treatment that claims to work for everyone or uses only testimonials as evidence; as compelling as these personal stories may be, they are not the same as scientific evidence. If there is scientific evidence, is it the result of one study, or several? Did those studies use a control group? The most trustworthy studies use a control group—people who did *not* receive the treatment being evaluated—to make sure other factors are not affecting the outcome. Ideally, the control subjects should receive a placebo, whether it's actually a sugar pill or a different form of therapy.

- **Is this treatment backed by objective experts?** The National Center for Complementary and Alternative Medicine is an affiliate of the National Institutes of Health that provides fact sheets to help educate consumers. The American Speech-Language-Hearing Association is the professional, scientific, and credentialing association for more than 123,000 members and affiliates who are speech therapists, audiologists, and scientists in the United States and abroad. What do they have to say about the therapy you're considering? Search at websites ncaam.nih.gov. and asha.org.

- **What does your gut say?** If you think a particular treatment sounds too good—or too weird—to be true, it may very well be. Talk to the professionals your child is working with and see what they think. Be particularly cautious when the treatment is an herb or medical procedure that could cause your child harm. If you are interested in trying a specific treatment—one that has a minimal risk—it may not hurt to try. Even if you're on the fence, the only harm that can come is to your wallet.

Diet-Based Therapies

Fish Oil/Essential Fatty Acids. Essential fatty acids (EFAs) are those fatty acids that are not produced by the body but are essential to the development and function of the brain as well as the normal growth of the muscles, nerves, and organs. And fish are just swimming in it. There are two types of essential fatty acids: Omega 6 and Omega 3.

Omega 6 fatty acids are common in the Western diet as they can be found in animal fats as well as in linoleic acid, which comprises the primary oil ingredient added to most processed foods and is found in commonly used cooking oils such as sunflower, safflower, and soybean oils.

Omega 3 fatty acids can be found in flaxseed oil, walnuts, dark green leafy vegetables, and cold-water fish including salmon, trout, sardines, mackerel, and cod—foods most likely to be lacking from the majority of mainstream diets.

Many studies extol the virtues of EFAs, and emerging evidence suggests it offers viable therapeutic benefits for treating depression, bipolar disorder, ADHD, postpartum depression, autism, heart disease, diabetes, and autoimmune disease.

In his book *The Omega-3 Connection*, Dr. Andrew L. Stoll writes, "Because the omega-3 oils are a major constituent of brain cell membranes and are converted to crucial brain chemicals, they are needed for normal nervous system function and seem to be involved in mood regulation, attention and memory, and psychosis."

What role does fish oil play in speech and language? One study from the University of British Columbia found a positive correlation between the amount of DHA—a particular type of Omega 3 fatty acid—in breast milk and language development in breast-fed infants. To date, any correlation between fish oil and speech or language disorders is strictly anecdotal. Some feel EFAs help with communication by improving a child's ability to focus, thus allowing him to better attend to the work being done in speech therapy.

Others feel the fish oil plays a more direct role in speech. As is the case with Laura's experience. When her son Cameron was diagnosed with apraxia, Laura started giving him a fish oil supplement. It took some experimenting, but after about two weeks of taking the right dosage "his speech exploded," she says. "He began putting sentences together and using words instead of gestures for things he wanted." Laura attributes her son's success to the EFAs. "Because of his sensory issues, Cameron doesn't eat a proper range of foods and wasn't getting any Omegas in his diet," she says. "I believe that once he started taking the fish oil, his brain was getting the nutrients it lacked and that is why we saw an improvement so quickly."

It is unlikely that EFA deficiency is the sole source of your child's language or speech problem. There is far more evidence that many conditions run in families. Still, there isn't much risk in giving your child fish oil supplements. Very few people experience side effects; those who do may have mild stomach upset or a fishy aftertaste, which can be minimized by taking small, divided doses with food and by using a high-quality product.

One way to introduce more EFAs into your child's diet is to have him eat more fish. However, you will need to be mindful of not going overboard. While both the Food and Drug Administration and the Environmental Protection Agency maintain that a well-balanced diet that includes a variety of fish can contribute to a child's proper growth and development, there is the issue, and possible risk, of mercury levels in seafood. Too much mercury may affect a child's developing nervous system. The FDA and EPA recommend that young children should avoid eating shark, swordfish, king mackerel, and tilefish because of their high levels of mercury. Fish with low levels of mercury include shrimp, canned light tuna, salmon, pollock, and catfish. Up to twelve ounces a week is recommended for an adult diet, so adjust accordingly for your child.

If this proves to be too much of a challenge, there are a variety of supplements on the market. If your child is too young to swallow a pill, there are also powder and liquid forms available. As with any supplement, talk with your child's pediatrician before giving him fish oil, and ask about the correct dosage. (If your pediatrician isn't knowledgeable about EFAs, you might want to consult a naturopath or a dietician.)

Gluten-Free/Casein-Free Diet. Following a wheat- and dairy-free diet is no walk in the park—packing a picnic certainly requires a lot of creativity. But many parents—especially those of children with autism—are reporting significant improvements in their children's speech once they remove these ingredients from their diet.

Gluten is a protein found in wheat, barley, rye, and oats; casein is a protein found in dairy products such as milk, ice cream, cheese, and yogurt. Once digested, these proteins are broken down into peptides. However, there are some children who are unable to properly digest these proteins, and when unbroken peptides enter the bloodstream they can have a negative effect on brain development. There is tremendous anecdotal evidence, and an increasing number of studies, to suggest that removing wheat and dairy from the diet of some children can yield positive results. Researchers at the University of Sunderland in the United Kingdom found that parents reported improvements in vocal and nonvocal communication, increased level of attention and concentration, and improved motor skills, among others, in their children with autism after three months of following a gluten-free diet. And in a review of twelve years' worth of studies on the effects of a gluten- and casein-free diet on children with autistic disorders, the results, as published in *Nutritional Neuroscience*, were pretty much the same across the board: reduction of autistic behavior, increased social and communication skills, and reappearance of autistic traits after the diet has been broken.

Following a gluten- and casein-free diet (GF/CF) requires considerable learning and planning, as well as strict adherence in order for you to see any improvements. Because there are far simpler approaches to helping your child's communication problems, the GF/CF diet shouldn't necessarily be your first line of defense. However, if your child has been diagnosed with autism or has other behavioral challenges, this may be a worthwhile protocol to try.

Sensory-Integration-Based Therapies

Craniosacral Therapy. Craniosacral therapy (CST) is a hands-on method that uses a soft touch—no greater than the weight of a nickel—to address restrictions of the body's central nervous system. The membranes and fluid that surround and protect the brain and spinal cord comprise the craniosacral system, which extends from the bones of the skull, face, and mouth (which make up the cranium) down to the tailbone (sacrum) area. CST practitioners—typically massage therapists, chiropractors, occupational therapists, and physical therapists—work to release problem areas and relieve undue pressure on the brain and spinal cord.

CST was first developed by osteopath John E. Upledger, a former clinical researcher who studied the existence and influence of the craniosacral system; the results of which helped him to develop craniosacral therapy.

Practitioners believe that CST aids the body's natural healing processes by releasing restrictions. "Imagine a garden hose across your driveway and someone parks on it," says Roy Desjarlais, vice president of clinical services and international affiliates at the Upledger Institute and a CST practitioner for twenty years. "You're watering your flowers and enough water gets through—but not enough for the flowers to thrive. We help facilitate moving the car off that garden hose so the water can be restored to the garden and the flowers can thrive."

Craniosacral therapy may play a role in improving sensory function, which can improve your child's ability to pay attention and process information—both of which positively affect speech and language skills. In addition, practitioners claim to address communication issues by working on specific cranial nerves. There are twelve pairs of cranial nerves that transit special information to and from the brain. Cranial nerve VIII (acoustic nerve) is involved with hearing, nerve X (vagus nerve) is involved in the ability to swallow and part of speech, and nerve XII (hypoglossal nerve) is mainly responsible for movement of the tongue.

It's important to bear in mind that researchers at the University of British Columbia conducted a systematic review of the scientific evidence on craniosacral therapy and had this to report: "The evidence that is available is of poor methodological quality, is highly variable, lacks consistency and does not allow any logical 'positive' conclusions regarding craniosacral therapy." Other studies show that physical therapists do not agree on the critical measurements in the procedures.

Upledger's philosophy puts less stock in scientific results and more in patient results because, he feels, it is not possible to control all of the variables in a study involving human subjects. Of course, positive patient outcomes should be measurable in scientifically designed studies. Whether or not you agree with this thinking should guide you in your decision to have your child undergo this therapy.

Hippotherapy. From the Greek word *hippos*, meaning horse, hippotherapy is literally "treatment with the help of a horse." This physical, occupational, and speech therapy method uses the movement of the horse to help those with impairments such as abnormal tone, impaired communication, and poor postural control; functional limitations such as gross motor skills, speech and language abilities, and behavioral and cognitive abilities; and medical conditions such as cerebral palsy, Down syndrome, and developmental delays. How? Practitioners believe the rhythmic movement of the horse contributes to improved muscle tone, balance, posture, coordination, strength, flexibility, and cognitive skills. The constant adjustments one makes for the horse's movements helps to improve sensorimotor integration.

Hippotherapy has been used more extensively with children with motor problems than with speech or language problems. So while there are studies that have demonstrated the effectiveness of this treatment in children with physical problems, such as cerebral palsy, there are no studies examining its impact on speech and language.

What does this mean for your child's speech and language skills? Some think that it will help. "The multi-dimensional movement of a well-cadenced horse facilitates all of the motor and sensory systems that produce speech," says Ruth Dismuke-Blakely, a New Mexico–based speech language pathologist and hippotherapy clinical specialist. "There also appears to be a strong overall arousal effect that helps to access more complex language structure and vocabulary."

According to Dismuke-Blakely, the movement of the horse has an impact on the underlying mechanics of speech production in several ways—postural control, respiratory control, motor control, and timing and rhythm—all of which play important roles in your child's ability to effectively produce speech.

Hippotherapy may also improve muscle tone, which is another key factor for communication. Low muscle tone, or hypotonia, can impair your child's rate of speech, voice quality, and the motor coordination necessary for movement of the tongue, lips, tongue, and palate, resulting in slow, slurred, or nasal speech.

Speech and language development is also dependent on a well-integrated sensory system. The constant adjustments riders must make for the horse's movements increases sensorimotor integration; this in turn may improve your child's ability to retrieve words, use proper syntax, organize his thoughts, and perform the necessary sequencing required for verbal communication.

> ## Parent to Parent
>
> "One of my daughter's therapists suggested hippotherapy and yes, I thought she was crazy. If trained, professional human beings could not get my daughter to eat, drink, and talk, how could a horse? But I was never so glad I was so wrong! Up until now, Francesca communicated with squeals, screams, and about five words only I understood. But once she started with the horse she immediately began to improve her balance and fine motor skills—and she was trying to talk!"
>
> —*Laura, mom to eight-year-old Francesca, apraxia and hypotonia*
> *(Baltimore, Maryland)*

While some consider hippotherapy to be an alternative therapy, those in the field take exception. "The animals are integrated into treatment just as one would use any other treatment activity, game, or reinforcement," wrote Beth L. Macauley, an assistant professor of communication disorders, now at the University of Tulsa, in a letter to *The ASHA Leader*. "They are incorporated within the ASHA scope of practice for speech-language pathology to help clients progress toward their communication goals."

Therapeutic Listening/Auditory Integration Therapy. Therapeutic listening, also known as auditory integration therapy, is a sensory-based treatment that according to practitioners, can help children who have difficulties with movement, auditory perception, language, and learning. It's based on the premise that listening to electronically altered music stimulates the neural pathways into the brain and helps the auditory and vestibular (balance) systems.

Children listen, through headphones, to carefully selected music in which the sound frequencies are electronically modulated, or distorted, for a prescribed amount of time each day. Proponents believe the brain becomes trained to filter out low frequencies of sounds and tune in higher frequencies, such as the sounds that characterize human speech. They report that when coupled with sensory integration therapy, therapeutic listening can improve your child's attention, self-regulation, postural control, motor control, and communication, among other areas.

The origins of this treatment are steeped in the works of ear, nose, throat specialists Alfred Tomatis and Guy Berard, as well as sound engineer Ingo Steinbach, each of whom has a method named for him. A key principle of the *Tomatis Method* is that listening plays a fundamental role in language, and that one's voice can only produce what one's ear can hear. Berard believed that hypersensitive hearing causes auditory processing problems. He developed a different method of filtering sound and used pop music rather than the classical used by Tomatis, known as *Auditory Integration Training*. Steinbach followed with the *SAMONAS Method* (Spectrally Activated Music of Optimal NAtural Structure), in which the choice of music is based on the principles of music therapy and includes classical music as well as nature sounds.

Although these therapies are in widespread use, their effectiveness has been called into question. Some doctors report their patients responded negatively to the treatment. Researchers at Northeastern University and Massachusetts Institute of Technology studied the device used to process the music and found the sound levels to be potentially harmful to one's hearing. And after reviewing Berard's Auditory Integration Therapy (the most commonly used therapeutic listening program in the United States), the American Speech-Language-Hearing Association published a technical report declaring that "this method did not meet scientific standards for efficacy and safety that would justify its inclusion as a mainstream treatment" for communication, behavioral, emotional, or learning disorders. In addition, the American Academy of Audiology, the American Academy of Pediatrics, and the Educational Audiology Association all concurred that auditory integration therapy should be considered an experimental procedure.

ONE THERAPEUTIC INTERVENTION DOES NOT FIT ALL

Remember, not all kids will respond to a particular treatment in the same way. Or at all. Whatever complementary therapy you may choose to try, get as much information on it as you can before starting something new. Make sure there's no risk to your child. Then, give it a reasonable amount of time before deciding it's not right for your child.

Some parents prefer to try one treatment at a time in order to assess what works and what doesn't. Others may try several all at once in hope of making faster progress. There is no right or wrong way to proceed.

"It's hard to say just how much the alternative therapies have helped," says Ann Marie, mom to Jenna. "You don't know if it's the new thing you added that worked, the traditional therapy, the combination, or if your child is just having a developmental spurt. We decided to stop analyzing everything. We still try new therapies, but we don't worry about which one is working—as long as Jenna is improving and we aren't doing anything that could be harmful."

To cover, in-depth, all the different complementary treatments available for speech and language disorders would require not a chapter, but an entire book. So if you're interested in pursuing any of the therapies discussed here, go online and do some research. Look for reputable and objective sources of information. Talk with other parents who have gone this route. Be sure to consult your child's pediatrician, neurologist, speech therapist, or other professional who is working with your child. And most of all, use your knowledge of your child, awareness of your own situation, and your own good judgment as you make decisions about which complementary and alternative therapies you may want to try.

8

Dealing with the Diagnosis: The Impact on Your Child, as Well as Your Marriage, Family, and Job

It took Dave an hour before he could bring himself to tell me what had happened.

It was well past nine o'clock—and Max's bedtime—when Dave went to check on him. Max was asking for "more milk" and although willing to oblige, Dave knew the importance of having Max use all his words. So he asked Max for the whole sentence, "I want more milk." Dave had to model each word for Max to repeat back. When they were done, Max told him, "It's hard."

I burst into tears as Dave relayed the story.

"Why didn't you tell me as soon as you were finished with him?" I asked.

"I didn't think I could tell you without crying," he said through his own tears.

It broke our hearts to realize that Max was very much aware of his struggle to speak. For so many months, despite his moments of frustration, we thought he was OK. Speech therapy had always been fun for him, and he'd never complained about going. His disorder never got in the way of his making friends. And he enjoyed every minute of preschool. This was our first indication that he was suffering emotionally.

After Dave and I calmed down, I went to talk with Max. I had no idea how much he would understand, but I felt the need to address what happened. I told him all the things my mom had drilled into me in my moments of frustration and failure over the years.

"Max," I said, "I know it's hard for you to talk sometimes and I want you to know I think you're doing great and I'm very proud of you. You're trying very hard and that's all that matters. If it's too hard to talk sometimes, that's OK."

His little voice responded, "OK, Mama," his standard response to much of what I say. I know he heard me, but did he understand? Did he know what the word "proud" means?

A speech or language disorder can affect far more than your child's ability to speak; it can affect every aspect of your child's life, including his behavior, mental health, and educational career. The day-to-day challenges of raising a child who can't clearly communicate can be a significant stress on your own mental health. Your other children may feel an imbalance in the family dynamics. Spouses who disagree about treatment or who have different ways of coping may feel added strain on their marriage. Careers are often put on hold.

This chapter will address the impact having a child with a speech or language problem has on all these areas. Let's start with how the diagnosis affects your child.

YOUR CHILD

Multiple studies report that communication impairment is linked to other disabilities, such as delays in reaching other developmental milestones, literacy difficulties, psychiatric diagnoses, and behavioral problems. In the July 2000 issue of *Developmental Medicine and Child Neurology*, researchers conducted neurological exams for seventy-two children with language impairment and eighty-two typically developing peers. Abnormalities were found in 70 percent of the children with language impairment, compared to only 22 percent of the control children. According to the study, "These findings suggest that developmental learning impairment is not an isolated finding but is indicative of more widespread nervous system dysfunction."

It sounds scary, I know. You have enough information to process as it is without being told your child could have additional problems. But the good news is that the earlier these problems can be identified, the greater chance your child has of responding to therapy.

Behavior

Children who struggle with speech and language may behave in ways that cause parents concern. Some kids turn their frustration outward and this can take the form of aggression or inattention, for example. Those who turn their feelings inward may demonstrate signs of anxiety or depression.

A study in the *Journal of the American Academy of Child and Adolescent Psychiatry* found that based on parent and teacher reports, 50 percent of children with speech and language problems showed behavioral problems in comparison with 12 percent of children without speech and language problems.

This does not mean that speech and language impairments *cause* behavioral problems. It's possible that both the communication and the behavioral issues stem from the same underlying cause. Researchers at Columbia University suggest that left-brain abnormalities may underlie both language impairment and behavior problems in boys. However, at the University of Minnesota, researchers believe that it is environmental factors, rather than neurodevelopmental ones, that predict antisocial behavior in adolescents.

Does this mean your child will have behavioral problems? Well, all kids are different. And how they respond to their communication challenges will vary, depending on their personality and the support they receive. Some will respond to their inability to express their thoughts with frustration. They may yell, become aggressive, and throw temper tantrums the likes of which you've never seen. Max became so exasperated he would hit his head against the floor or wall.

Others may withdraw and stop communicating. There have been times when in my efforts to understand what Ari was explaining to me, she would tire and end the conversation with a "never mind."

"Cameron is working on his reading, but he gets frustrated very quickly and will start to cry," says mom Laura. "The behavior problems start when his level of self-confidence goes down because he is struggling with something. Then, it's almost as though he gets depressed. We have to very gently bring him around."

Some kids who lack control over their ability to communicate become controlling over everything else in their lives, which can lead to acting out if their demands are not met. Max not only preferred that I brush his teeth or read him his bedtime story, there were times he would become agitated if I wasn't the one to put in his video.

Kids who have trouble talking or understanding may act out in the classroom. Others choose to observe rather than participate because it's easier for them. They may hesitate to speak in class for fear of embarrassment. They may have difficulty making friends. They may not be able to tell you about their day at school.

One of the most common coexisting problems is difficulty with memory, according to Sally Bloch, Ph.D., a clinical psychologist in West Bloomfield, Michigan. "Memories tend to be organized using language," says Bloch. "Without language to organize incoming experiences, accessing these memories when a similar situation arises becomes haphazard at best. The child may seem to know something one day, and then lose that knowledge the next. Parents might also have great difficulty establishing patterns of behavior. For example, even though the morning routine may be exactly the same every day, the child may behave as though it is new each morning—causing considerable frustration for the parents."

Some children's frustrations manifest in such extreme behaviors that it's not uncommon for professionals to misdiagnosis their speech or language disorder for something else, such as autism or ADHD. Often these behaviors start to resolve once the speech or language issue is identified and treated.

How You Can Help

- **Don't panic.** "I have seen many parents who are so anxious about the language delay that it robs them of fully enjoying their child," says Bloch. "Every birthday becomes tinged with grief and worry that the child has not yet caught up to his peers." I know it's hard—and I'm not always able to follow this advice myself—but panicking doesn't help. Get it out of your system by talking with a friend or writing in a journal, and move on to more constructive ways of helping your child.

- **Be empathetic.** Imagine that you are alone in a foreign country and you don't speak the language—it's frightening, stressful, and isolating. This may be just how your child is feeling. Remind her that she is still learning how to talk and that you are going to help her.

- **Don't let her get too frustrated.** In their book, *The Late Talker: What to Do If Your Child Isn't Talking Yet*, authors Marilyn C. Agin, M.D., Lisa F. Geng, and Malcolm J. Nicholl offer this advice: "There's a breaking point that most parents have to discover the hard way—the number of times they can incorrectly guess what their child said before he becomes frustrated and tearful. They learn it's best to divert the child's attention before reaching that point."

- **Be a parent, not another speech therapist.** While it's important to encourage your child to use his words—and use them correctly—you need to recognize when your child has had enough prompting and drilling. Don't let your determination to help your child's progress override her need for you to simply be her parent.

- **Try alternative methods of communicating.** Teach your child some basic signs, such as those for *more, help, eat,* and *drink* to reduce his frustration. Have him help you make picture books or posters he can use to express his needs; have separate books or posters for different categories such as food, toys, family members, and places to visit.

- **Remind her of all the things she does well.** It could be drawing, taking care of the dog, or being a good friend. Remind her that everyone has something they need help with whether it's glasses for poor vision or a tutor for math. "I have really involved Brennan cognitively in this process by talking to him frankly about his speech differences and encouraging him to work harder because of them," says mom Cara. "I tell him, 'Brennan, you know you need help with your talking. It's hard for you to be understood by others sometimes. That's frustrating and it's not fair. I'm sorry it's so hard for you. All of us have something that's difficult for us.' It seems to help him understand his responsibility in speech therapy."

- **Find ways to interact with your child that don't require talking.** Take a walk together, create something with Play-Doh, bake cookies, plant a vegetable garden, give her a backrub, have a water balloon fight. By finding ways to enjoy each other's company—without the need for language—you reinforce your bond and let your child know you love and accept her, regardless of her communication problem.

- **Support your child socially.** Make sure he has opportunities to play with peers and develop relationships with them. Sign him up for a parent-toddler class. Join a local playgroup. Spend time at the park. If he's old enough, enroll him in preschool for two or three mornings a week. You may be busy with appointments and therapy sessions, but it's important to make the time to not only allow your child to develop his social skills, but to simply be a kid and have fun.

- **Review Chapter 9 for strategies for your child's specific diagnosis.**

Mental Health

Many researchers have found that a child's inability to express him or herself or understand others can be associated with serious emotional and behavioral problems. In fact, several studies suggest that children with psychiatric disorders have previously undiagnosed language impairments.

In her study, "Early language impairment and young adult delinquent and aggressive behavior," published in the *Journal of Abnormal Child Psychology*, E. B. Brownlie identified four possible correlations between language impairment and what she termed "late adolescent delinquency symptoms":

- **School functioning.** Children with language impairment may have a more difficult time functioning at school. "Now that Payton is five, the speech problem is starting to affect him at school," says mom Kelly. "I know the gym teacher thinks he has a behavior issue, but it is nearly impossible for him to understand her speaking in a gym with any noise going on." Negative school experiences may play an important role in the development of antisocial behavior in boys. In some cases, such negative school experiences may be attributed to poor academic performance—which could be an indication of a learning disability.
- **Executive function.** Also known as self-regulation, this is the cognitive ability that allows us to plan, monitor, and change our own behavior. Kids rely on self-directed speech—you know it as talking to yourself—to consider possibilities and make decisions. But this important function can be compromised in a child with language difficulties; if it's compromised to the point that your child's daily functioning is impaired, it's possible he may have ADHD.
- **Social life.** Because language plays a key role in social interactions, children with language impairment may not interact with their peers as often as other children. They may find themselves in situations in which the need to communicate exceeds their ability to do so. "I do think Decker's language difficulties affected his ability to connect with other kids," says mom Frith. "Often he would just shut down or give up whatever toy he had without asserting himself." It's not uncommon for these kids to experience

social anxiety or to require help developing their social skills. At home, comprehension and expression difficulties may create an ongoing challenge to the parent-child relationship, resulting in fewer positive interactions.

- **Theory of mind.** Language impairment may interfere with your child's ability to understand the feelings of others and affect what Brownlie calls their "social competence and moral development." At the far end of the spectrum, this could lead to a child being diagnosed with oppositional defiant disorder.

Children with speech or language difficulties may also have trouble regulating their emotions. Those who internalize their emotions are at high risk of depression and anxiety, which can take the form of general anxiety, obsessive-compulsive disorder, separation anxiety, social anxiety, or selective mutism. Kids who externalize their emotions may feel anger and frustration and may experience mood swings in which they rapidly move in and out of feelings of anger.

None of this is intended to panic you, but rather, to make you aware of possible risks. Will your child have a mental health disorder? It may be hard to determine right now. But by having this information, you will be better prepared to identify—and treat—any future problems.

How You Can Help

- **Put him in a social language class.** Also known as social skills class, or less therapeutic sounding names such as friendship circle, these groups may be run by a speech pathologist, child psychologist, or both. This is a safe environment for your child to learn much needed skills such as taking turns in conversation, working with others, thinking about another person's feelings, and finding constructive ways to express negative feelings.
- **Sign her up for something fun.** She can develop and practice her social skills when she's participating in something with other kids her age. Try a parent-toddler class, music class, book club, soccer

team, pottery class, or anything else that interests her. Depending on your child's needs, you may want to fill the instructor in on her speech or language limitations.

- **Read social stories.** Although this therapeutic technique was originally designed to help children with autism, you can use this simple tool to teach your child how to behave in special situations, perform specific activities, and respond appropriately when expressing negative feelings.

- **Consult a child psychologist.** If your child exhibits any behavior that causes you concern, you have nothing to lose by talking with a professional. The information and insight you'll gain will either put your mind at ease or give you a head start on addressing a coexisting problem.

Literacy

Many experts argue that a language disorder is at the core of learning disabilities. According to their book, *Diagnosis and Management of Learning Disabilities: An Interdisciplinary/Lifespan Approach*, authors Frank R. Brown, Elizabeth H. Aylward, and Barbara K. Keogh wrote that in 1980, one researcher predicted that "the language-delayed preschooler of today may well become the learning-disabled student of tomorrow." The authors point toward the growing body of evidence that supports this prediction and suggest that many of these children do not "outgrow" these problems; that "simple" delays in communications may, in fact, be stable predictors of later learning disabilities.

Numerous studies support the notion that spoken language is a necessary foundation for the development of reading and writing skills. The fact that spoken and written language share a reciprocal relationship is further supported simply by the existence of ASHA's guidelines on the "Roles and Responsibilities of Speech-Language Pathologists Related to Reading and Writing in Children and Adolescents."

"Language comprehension really affects every single subject in school," says mom Terri. "Elena used to at least have a little relief in math. But the curriculum has been changed to include writing in every single subject, including math, which is positively sadistic for kids who have language problems. This year, she even has to keep a journal for band. It's tough."

Speech and language researchers have well established that children who have difficulty forming speech are at significant risk of delays in their development of phonological awareness and literacy skills. But phonological awareness is more than just the ability to match a letter with its sound; according to Joy Stackhouse, a registered speech and language therapist and professor of human communication sciences at the University of Sheffield in the United Kingdom, it is many related skills:

- Recognition and production of rhyme
- Identification of number of syllables
- Sound to word matching (identifying the beginning sound of a word)
- Word to word matching (determining if two words begin with the same sound)
- Sound deletion (identifying words once a sound has been removed)
- Sound segmentation (identifying the individual sounds that comprise a word)

When you stop to think about the many steps necessary for a child to read and spell, it's easy to see the connection between speech and literacy difficulties.

"When spelling a new word, children have to be able to segment the word into its sounds before they can attach the appropriate letters, and when reading an unfamiliar word, they have to be able to decode the printed letters back to sounds," writes Stackhouse in her paper, "Phonological awareness: Connecting speech and literacy problems."

Researchers in the United Kingdom found that children with persisting speech problems at age six years, nine months were vulnerable to deficits in reading-related processes. Those with phonological disorders were also at high risk of reading difficulties. Another group following two-to-six-year-old "late talkers" found that although the majority had outgrown their language deficits by age four, they demonstrated delays in academic readiness at ages five and six.

Now, I wasn't privy to any of this information when my kids were being diagnosed or treated. But I knew from what I had read about apraxia that they would potentially have trouble learning how to read and write. And I began to look at every developmental step—or lack thereof—through this apraxia screen.

When Max was four years old, I remember being concerned about his messy handwriting. I explained to his pre-k teachers that Max might have trouble with this because of his apraxia diagnosis. They kindly explained that Max's handwriting looked very much like that of his classmates. "The kids tend to hold the pencil too tightly," Mrs. T. explained. "If you do that, it makes your hand shake."

With Ari, I never had a chance to worry about her literacy skills. She was learning to read almost a year earlier than Max. Her pre-k teacher told me she was the only child in her class who knew all twenty-six sounds of the alphabet. And Ari's idea of fun has always been sitting with a pencil and some paper and writing notes, often along the lines of "Dear Mom, please may I have a puppy for my Strawberry Shortcake?"

Just because your child has a speech or language problem doesn't mean he will also have literacy problems. But if he does, the good news is that these delays can often be identified during the preschool years. By keeping an eye out for such problems, and providing intervention at an early age, your child may resolve any potential difficulties before he starts kindergarten. Even if he doesn't, you'll be in a better position to help your child and advocate for the necessary supports in school.

How You Can Help

- **Show your child the value of reading and writing.** Of course you should read to your child every day, but you can further motivate him to read and write by connecting these skills to activities he enjoys. Read a recipe together to make his favorite cake. Check the newspaper to find out what time the latest Disney flick is playing. Have him write a list for the supermarket; once you get there, have him cross off each item from the list as you put it in the cart. Ask him to find the exit you need on the highway.

- **Balance homework with fun.** Starting in the first grade, reading will be part of your child's homework. Find a time to do it when there's no time pressure. Pick a comfortable spot in the house. Encourage your child to read, but don't push her to the point where she shuts down and refuses to try.

- **Read collaboratively.** Let your child choose the book he'll read to you. As soon as he starts to struggle, provide the word. Yes, ideally you want him to put in the time and effort to sound out the letters. But if he's easily frustrated, providing the word right away will allow you to bypass a potential tantrum or shutdown and you can continue with your reading time.

- **Label items around the house.** Index cards work well in identifying things in your home such as *refrigerator, stove, door, chair,* to help your child make the connection between objects and the written words that represent them. Once your child has learned how to read these words, have her put them in a special box and start a collection of words she can read. Add to the collection by making more index cards of words that are of particular interest to your child (Max's cards included *Darth, Vader, saber,* and *Luke*). Make a set of cards for an upcoming trip to the zoo, and have your child match the cards with the animals you see.

- **Have reasonable expectations.** Before you jump to conclusions—as I have on more than one occasion—that your child's difficulty with reading or writing is related to his communication problem, talk with the teacher. There is a wide range of abilities in these areas, especially in the earlier grade levels. Your child's teacher will be able to put your concerns in perspective by explaining grade-level expectations and discussing possible support services at school.

- **Don't be afraid to consult a reading specialist or psychologist.** If you still have concerns about your child's reading or writing abilities, remember, as with speech and language, early intervention is always best. A reading specialist or psychologist can test your child for a learning disability and, in the absence of one, make recommendations on how you can best support your child.

YOUR EMOTIONAL WELL-BEING

Let's see. We had severe behavioral problems with Max, learned of his apraxia diagnosis and his need for intensive speech therapy, decided I should quit my job, fought with the insurance company over coverage—fought with my husband over many things—tried to keep my career going, worried about Max's future, and eventually learned that Ari had the same diagnosis. Yeah, I guess you could say my emotional well-being had been thoroughly challenged.

And I wasn't the only one. Researchers in Germany thought the emotional state of mothers such as myself was significant enough to merit a study, "Anxiety and depression in mothers of speech impaired children." The results of the study indicated that 11 percent of the mothers of children with speech impairment met criteria for depression compared to only 2½ percent of mothers in the control group. The reasons for this were, to me, not the least bit surprising. Researchers found that mothers:

- Typically take on a larger part of the extra care a child with speech or language problems requires.
- Often have to give up their job and personal interests in order to do so.
- Feel added strain because of their responsibility of supporting speech therapy at home.

- Are concerned about the child's future and whether the child will be socially accepted.
- Worry that the communication impairment may lead to the development of other disorders such as hyperactivity, oppositional behavior, and emotional disturbances.

Still, it's important to point out that although 11 percent of the mothers of children with speech impairment met the criteria for depression, the majority of mothers did not.

For me, the feelings of depression were situational. There was the initial wave of feeling overwhelmed upon learning of Max's—and then Ari's—problem. But after I had some time to simply *feel*—loss, frustration, anxiety—and process the information, the need to get my children help overrode everything else. As their speech improved, so, too, did my mood. There were still moments when I was reminded of their impairment—a friend's verbally precocious child; Max being shut out from some chatty girls playing "school"—and I would be taken back to those early days when we first were given the news of Max's disorder and I'd have to dig my way out of it again.

"We were already in the trenches of therapy with my daughter when my son was diagnosed," says mom Mary. "That was when we realized the kids had some real issues. We were depressed; not a day would go by that I wouldn't think about how things were different for us. But now we understand what apraxia is, we're armed with knowledge, and we're able to find ways to work with it. We don't dwell on it. Some days go by and I don't think about the differences all that much anymore. You have to move forward and keep learning and working."

The Five Stages of Grief

People feel grief in many situations other than the death of a loved one. The loss of a job. A divorce. A move to another state. When you realize your child has a problem, you may also feel a loss. Loss of a future you had hoped for your child that she may not have.

It is perfectly normal to mourn the loss of a "normal" child, and it is not uncommon for parents to experience some, if not all, of the stages of grief first identified by psychiatrist Elisabeth Kubler-Ross (sometimes in order, sometimes not) in these situations:

Denial. Parents who suspect something is not quite right about their child's communication but continue to wait and see if he improves on his own are likely experiencing denial. Denial can delay getting a much-needed evaluation. Even after a diagnosis has been made, parents in denial may question the competence of the person administering the tests. They may blame daycare providers or teachers for not providing their child with the appropriate environment and stimulation. Or they may argue with their spouse that their child is being pushed to do something he's not ready for yet. "My husband had some trouble in the beginning accepting that anything was wrong with our son, but he has seen the difference with speech therapy," says mom Pamela. "Once he saw that there was, in fact, a problem he was more than willing to do whatever it took. We now share the burden by alternating who takes Russell to speech therapy."

Anger. Some parents respond to the news of their child's speech or language problem with anger. They may lash out at any number of people including the professional who offers her assessment, the spouse who has a family history of communication disorders, or well-intentioned loved ones who question the validity of the diagnosis.

Bargaining. Parents with a faith in God may find themselves trying to make a deal and promising to do everything in their power to help their child as long as she'll be fine in the end. Others may bargain with themselves thinking, "If I just put him in speech therapy, everything will be fine."

Depression. The uncertainty of your child's future, the overwhelming feelings at learning of his problem, and the powerlessness and vulnerability you may experience may all contribute to feelings of depression. Some mothers may have feelings of guilt if they believe they may have done something during pregnancy to create the problem. "When my son was first diagnosed with severe apraxia at twenty-five months I was devastated," says mom Dee. "I cried myself to sleep at night worrying about whether he'd ever live a 'normal' life, be able to speak clearly enough to be understood, or require an assistive communication device." Bear in mind that depression can manifest itself in many different ways; if you're feeling irritable, agitated, and short-tempered for a length of time, you could be experiencing some depression.

Acceptance. Accepting your child's disability comes after you've allowed yourself the time to feel your emotions and process all the information. Now you are in the best position to advocate for your child and get her the help she needs. "Once I got past the initial shock and pain, I moved into a very proactive phase of learning everything I could about the diagnosis," says mom Dee. "I stayed up nights learning, and I joined both Internet and local parent groups. This helped me feel more in control." Even after you've reached the acceptance stage, many parents report periodic feelings of anger, sadness, and depression. Mom Jennifer says it is sometimes difficult to hear her friends' children talk. "Although they are younger than Emily, they say some amazing things," says Jennifer. "I almost feel it necessary to say that my daughter is smart and special, too. Maybe even more so because she had to find other ways to make her needs known." For mom Rachel, each new evaluation or progress update is especially difficult. "I go through a mourning period that is a very private time for me," she says. "Only a parent of such a child could understand how the information affects you as a mother and your concerns for your child's educational, emotional, and social future."

Parent to Parent

"When my daughter was three years old, my friend thought I was just being overprotective when I told her that Francesca couldn't chew regular food. She used to tell me to just give my daughter her space and that she'll be fine. Behind my back she gave Francesca a cracker and I watched as she practically turned blue from choking. That was the end of our friendship."

> —*Laura, mom to eight-year-old Francesca, apraxia and hypotonia*
> *(Baltimore, Maryland)*

"My friends saw the glass as being half full. They didn't understand why I would be affected so much by my daughter's difficulties. They knew I was getting her the help she needed and they figured she'd be fine. It is just a very isolating process."

> —*Rachel, mom to seven-year-old Maya, expressive/receptive*
> *language disorder (Dobbs Ferry, New York)*

"I've met such wonderful people that I never would have met otherwise. Fellow parents of kids with various disabilities—both locally and online—all of these people have enriched my life so much that I truly feel in many ways the diagnosis was a blessing in disguise."

> —*Dee, mom to ten-year-old Adam, severe apraxia*
> *(Madison, Wisconsin)*

"We are constantly hearing about other parents who are in the same boat as us. It's sort of like being in a special club, where you celebrate each language milestone with your child because you know they worked so hard to get there."

> —*Frith, mom to three-year-old Decker, moderate-severe expressive*
> *language delay (Pleasant Hill, California)*

Parent to Parent

"I cope by handing everything off to my husband, along with the insurance card, and say, 'Here—you deal with this crap for a while.'"
—*Pamela, mom to two-and-a-half-year-old Russell, dysphagia, sensory integration disorder (Tulsa, Oklahoma)*

How to Cope

- **Realize you are not alone.** You are not the first parent whose child has been diagnosed with a speech or language problem. Seek out other parents like yourself. Those who have been down this same path will prove to be a wealth of information and compassion. Your speech therapist may host a parent support group. Or, look online for support. Try the message boards at speechville.com or join the Listserv at apraxia-kids.org. (Even if your child doesn't have apraxia, you will find a wealth of relevant information on the site as well as from your fellow parents on the Listserv.)
- **Talk to your spouse.** Couples don't always react to stressful situations in the same way. If you're feeling emotional and your partner copes by spending hours on the Internet looking for information, you may not feel supported. Talk about your feelings and what you need from each other.
- **If your emotions are too overwhelming, consider talking to a therapist.** You'll be in a better position to take care of your child if you take care of yourself first.
- **Know that your feelings of love for your child may be overshadowed by feelings of grief or distress—and that's normal.** According to Laura E. Marshak, Ph.D. and Fran Pollock Prezant, M.Ed., authors of *Married with Special-Needs Children: A Couples' Guide to Keeping Connected*, "Understand that grief doesn't mean you don't love your child. Grief over the loss of the child you dreamed of does not invalidate any love you have for your newly diagnosed child."

- **Learn the terms.** You'll be hearing lots of new terminology from doctors and speech pathologists. If you don't understand something, ask. If you have trouble with their explanation, ask again. Or research it online. The more you understand, the better equipped you'll be to support your child's therapy.

- **Gather information.** Always get copies of your child's evaluations, progress reports, IEPs (more on what these are in Chapter 10), and all pertinent paperwork. Try to organize everything in an accordion folder or three-ring notebook. It's hard to process everything while you're in the middle of it. You may be in a better position to understand your child's condition once you're past the emotional stage, and you don't want to spend time trying to track down paperwork from a few months back.

- **Keep your job.** Some parents may find that the only way they can give their child the time and energy she needs is to leave their job. That was my experience, in the beginning. But it may be right for you to keep working. Staying in a job, according to researchers in Germany, allows mothers to focus on something other than their child; this may reduce the stress caused by having a child with a communication disability.

- **Use coping strategies that have worked for you in the past.** Whether it's exercising, getting a massage, treating yourself to a new book or CD, or indulging in the occasional pint of Häagen-Dazs chocolate chocolate chip, it's important that you take care of yourself and find outlets for your stress.

- **Appreciate the small moments.** Mom Pamela says, "Sometimes I have to just stop thinking about how worried I am about Russell, praying that he will be a normal child, that he will be even close to his older brother in intelligence, that he won't freak out during the hospital tests, that nothing happens to my husband because I almost can't deal with Russell by myself some days, praying that I'll be able to hear him speak intelligibly, if nothing else. And then, from the top of the stairs I hear, 'You're a princess, Mommy.' "

YOUR RELATIONSHIP

Children can be a strain on the best of relationships. There's the loss of private couple time, the constant exhaustion of attending to the child's every need, and of course, the universal debate about who's doing more around the house. Factor in a child who has special needs and the strain can feel even greater.

My conflicts with Dave usually revolved around who was doing more work. I wasn't resentful that I was the one responsible for taking the kids to their therapy sessions, working with them at home, maintaining contact with daycare providers and teachers, submitting bills to our insurance company and fighting for reimbursement, and reading everything about apraxia I could get my hands on. I didn't expect Dave to do any of these things. But I did expect him to unload the dishwasher every once in a while.

Researchers at the University of Wisconsin-Madison have found that compared to parents of children without special needs, marital disruption for parents of children with a developmental disability is more highly associated with the stress related to their parenting role.

Authors Laura E. Marshak and Fran Pollock Prezant caution parents raising children with special needs of the challenges you may experience:

- Establishing or reestablishing a bond despite the tendency of your child's disability to be all encompassing
- Accepting differences in emotional reactions to your child's problem
- Adjusting to roles that meet family needs in a way that feels fair and doesn't breed resentment
- Retaining the romance in your relationship and the ability to see each other as more than just parenting partners
- Developing a creative vision for the future and working as a team

Another area of stress between parents is what Marshak and Prezant refer to as "immersion vs. distraction" methods of coping. It's not uncommon for one partner to get immersed in the child's diagnosis, gathering as much information as possible. Such information is needed, of course, but the act of acquiring it is a coping strategy, allowing the parent "to gain a sense of control over a fearsome situation," according to the authors. Often their spouse, by contrast, finds distraction from the stressful situation by spending time with work, hobbies, or activities that take him or her outside the home. He or she may appear less involved with the child, but it's not for a lack of love; it's simply an attempt to avoid anxiety and reduce the impact of their child's problem. Both strategies are valid attempts for dealing with emotional distress, and in her years of practice as a psychologist, Marshak has seen far more couples in which "the husbands adopted a style that attempted to preserve normality and the wives were immersed in the disorder," she says.

"My husband and his family were much less proactive and often downplayed the significance—and even the existence—of my son's disability," says mom Dee. "My family and I were on top of things all the time. I felt like I was learning and doing while my husband was ignoring the problem."

It's important to note that the same University of Wisconsin researchers who found more marital conflict in couples who had a child with a disability, also determined that most parents are successful in accommodating their child's special needs. These families are able to make necessary adjustments, such as moms cutting back on work and both parents sharing childcare duties with other family members. "There is no doubt that there are increased sources of stress for parents who have children with significant disabilities," says Fran Pollock Prezant. "But we found that stress does not always equate with dysfunctionality of the family or marriage and that some families thrive and become stronger."

"The diagnosis was a strain on my marriage, due to my resentment of having to sacrifice so much while my husband didn't sacrifice anything. It created even more imbalance between our household and childcare duties than had previously existed. Eventually, as the diagnosis became less of an issue and more of a routine, those feelings of resentment faded. It doesn't really affect our marriage anymore."
    —Dee, mom to ten-year-old Adam, severe apraxia (Madison, Wisconsin)

"Payton was our first child. What his diagnosis did was delay the arrival of our second child. I didn't think it was fair to him—or to a new baby—to make any changes to our family until I felt that we had a handle on his speech."
    —Kelly, mom to five-year-old Payton, receptive and expressive language delay, semantic and pragmatic language issues (Milwaukee, Wisconsin)

How to Cope

- **Acknowledge that you and your partner will deal with emotions differently.** According to Marshak and Prezant, it's important to accept the differences in your coping styles without drawing conclusions about what it means. "For example, you may feel distressed by your partner's lack of overt emotion," they write in their book Married with Special-Needs Children, "but it may simply represent his or her attempt to cope, to conform to gender role expectations, or to keep from falling apart emotionally."
- **Have your spouse receive information from someone other than you.** This is most important when your spouse is in denial of your child's problem. When one partner doesn't attend therapy sessions or talk with doctors, that partner may dismiss the information you relay because he or she is removed from the situation. "It is not unusual for spouses to accept the veracity of information they

have heard from their partner only after hearing it from a professional," write Marshak and Prezant.

- **Give yourself a break from parenting.** Having adult time together is crucial to feeling connected—especially when your child has special needs. You'll feel more comfortable leaving your child if you tell your sitter about his speech or language problem and how she can best communicate with him. If you have trouble finding an appropriate sitter, try contacting the local university's early education, child psychology, or speech pathology departments for a referral—college students are always in need of extra cash and you know you'll get someone who loves children.

- **Give yourself a break from each other.** Yes, your time together is most likely limited. But it will be far more enjoyable time together if you both have other social and emotional outlets. That means attending your monthly book club meetings or weekly tennis games. The best way you can help your child is by maintaining a healthy marriage. And you can keep your marriage healthy by pursuing your individual interests and taking a break from your role as parent.

- **Don't forget to laugh.** Humor has been found to reduce tension, encourage intimacy, and according to one study in *European Psychiatry*, serve as a positive coping strategy used by families of children with disabilities. And while I have cried many tears over Max and Ari, their communication challenges have also provided wonderful comic relief. I can still remember the time I picked Max up from daycare and he told me, "Me Carrie sex." I knew that couldn't be right, so I asked him to repeat it. "Me Carrie sex hee haw hee haw," he said. He was waving his hands over his ears, but I still had no idea what he was trying to tell me. A few more "hee haws" and it finally clicked. "Max," I asked him, "Did you watch *Shrek* with Carrie today?" "Yeah!" he said, and continued to make what I failed to recognize as donkey sounds.

- **Keep the faith.** Whether you have faith in a higher power, or simply in your child, it's important to try to maintain a positive outlook. Some parents turn to their religious faith for a source of strength and comfort. "The main thing that has gotten me and my husband through this is our faith in God," says mom Mary. "We're no Pollyannas . . . we certainly have gone through various stages of mourning over the loss of 'normalcy.' We do not claim to understand why God allows disabilities to happen, but we have faith that there is a reason. We believe that raising a child with a disability of any kind is an honor and a calling."

- **Turn to family and friends for support.** Having people you can turn to, whether it's a shoulder to cry on or a last minute sitter, can make a world of difference in coping with your child's challenges. According to an article in *Sensory Integration Focus,* "Mothers who felt supported by their spouses, their friends, or members of their extended families had higher levels of satisfaction in their marriages and more positive adaptation to having a child with a disability." Mom Frith felt fortunate that her extended family offered more than just moral support. "My parents and sisters asked for a printout of the sign language signs we were teaching Decker and they made an effort to use them," she says. "They also asked if there were certain strategies we were using, or things we didn't want them to do, so they could help support our efforts. It was great knowing that the things we were working on with Decker were being reinforced when he visited his relatives."

YOUR OTHER CHILDREN

Although she didn't know it, there was a time when Ari was getting the short end of the stick.

When Max was an infant, I was able to breast-feed, albeit in conjunction with formula, for four full months. With Ari, I lasted only two weeks. It's not that I didn't want to nurse; it's just that it was extremely difficult to put baby to breast when there was a two-year-old already latched on to my hip. Ari didn't care who held her, fed her, or changed her perpetually poopy diapers as long as it was

Respite Care

Depending on your family's particular needs, and the nature of your child's impairment, you may want to consider respite care. Private companies are available for a fee, but there are organizations that offer services on a sliding scale basis or free of charge, depending on your state's eligibility requirements. For more information, contact one of these organizations:

Arch National Respite Network and Resource Center
archrespite.org
(919) 490-5577
The site's respite locator allows you to search for service providers by state, child's age, and nature of the impairment.

National Association of Councils on Developmental Disabilities
nacdd.org
(703) 739-4400
Visit the site's council directory for a state-by-state listing of councils on developmental disabilities.

The Friendship Circle
friendshipcircle.com
(248) 788-7878 ext. 211
Although this organization is affiliated with the Chabad-Lubavitch movement, a branch of Hasidic Judaism, its services are available to all in the community. This unique program matches teenage volunteers with children with special needs in order to give parents a much needed break. There are thirty-three locations in twelve states—plus Canada and Australia—and more being formed.

all getting done. Max, on the other hand, constantly demanded not just any attention, but specifically mine. This was before his apraxia diagnosis, when Max's inability to communicate made him prone to some world-class meltdowns. He didn't have the words to tell us what he wanted, and we were equally ill-equipped to handle the behavior that ensued. We became slaves to his screaming. And hard as it was helping him through these tantrums before Ari was born, it became even more challenging once I was hooked up to a breast pump.

So it was I who continued to pour Max's milk, join him on his pound-a-ball toy, brush his teeth, read *Jamberry* and *Mama, Do You Love Me?*, scratch his back, watch Elmo videos, kiss the boo-boos, and sing three different alphabet songs every night. I did all these things not because I had a husband who couldn't or wouldn't, but because I had a son who communicated that I was the only one who could do these things. His tears and yelling and outstretched hands said only I possessed the necessary qualifications.

So I handed Ari over to Dave. Over and over and over again. It was he, in those early months, who fed her and played with her and comforted her in the middle of the night. While I was busy giving Max what he wanted, what he needed, Dave did the same for Ari. And slowly, unexpectedly, she became his.

My need to take care of Max, to figure out how to help him, superseded everything—including my ability to bond with my new daughter. It would be many months into the future, when a rotavirus kept me and Ari homebound for several days, that our bond would finally form.

It's a challenge—for any parent—to maintain a balance between our kids. It's an even bigger challenge for the parent of a child with a special need, such as a speech or language disorder. All too easily, we are consumed by the problem. What is it called? How do we treat it? What can I do? Will my child be OK? And in our attempts to make life easier for our communication-challenged child, we may unintentionally make things a bit harder for our other kids.

Since Ari was an infant, she wasn't aware of the imbalance I had unintentionally created. But your older children will certainly be aware of the extra time and attention their sibling receives. And it's likely they'll experience a range of emotions, all of which are normal.

Confusion and Worry

Learning your child has a speech or language problem can be a confusing time for parents. So imagine how your other children might be feeling. Try as you might to keep conversations about your child's diagnosis between you and your spouse, kids have a way of picking up on the emotions of the household. If you're worried, they know it; they just might not know why. If you don't explain to them what the doctor and therapy appointments are about, they may imagine something far worse than their brother or sister having a speech or language disorder. Avoid any undue anxiety by explaining, in age-appropriate terms, the type of problem their sibling is experiencing. ("Dana has trouble speaking clearly." "Kevin needs to learn how to use his voice the right way." "Sometimes Connor doesn't understand all the words you say to him.") Explain how the speech therapist is helping your child. If possible, allow siblings to observe a session so they don't feel in the dark. Let them ask the SLP questions.

Jealousy and Anger

Your children may understand their sibling's problem and why you're giving them extra time and attention—but don't expect them to think it's fair. After all, they're still kids, and any feelings of jealousy or anger they may have are perfectly normal. Talk to them about the extra time your one child requires right now. Validate their feelings. And be sure to make time for all your children. Attend their soccer games. Ask about their friends. Help them study for their math test. Treating your children fairly doesn't necessarily mean equally—not when you have a child with needs that require extra time and attention. Between your job, household responsibilities, your kids' extracurricular activities, and the time spent traveling to and from speech therapy, you may only have fifteen minutes a day to give each of your other children your undivided attention. That's OK. Give it to them. Make sure they know they're as much a priority as your other child. It doesn't take equal time to assure them that they are equally loved.

Embarrassment and Guilt

As an adult, you're likely to find comfort in talking with your friends about your child's problem and your feelings. But your children may have trouble finding the words to express themselves. They may struggle with conflicting emotions and not know that it's OK to talk about it. Let them know that whatever embarrassment they may sometimes feel about their sibling doesn't negate their feelings of love. Sometimes kids feel guilty for losing their patience with their sibling or because they don't share the same problem. Allow your children the opportunity to talk about these feelings, and assure them what they're feeling is perfectly normal.

Protectiveness and Pride

Fortunately, along with all the negative feelings, siblings also experience many positive feelings—and develop important traits. Studies have shown that children who had a sibling with a disability had higher levels of empathy and altruism, increased tolerance for dif-

Parent to Parent

"The diagnosis helped our older son understand what was wrong with his brother, and in that way it helped him have a concrete reason why we needed to pay more attention to our apraxic son."

—*Dee, mom to ten-year-old Adam, severe apraxia (Madison, Wisconsin)*

ferences, an increased sense of maturity and responsibility, and pride in their sibling's accomplishments. Your other children can become additional advocates for your child, especially at school when you're not around. And if they are interested in helping their brother or sister with communication, show them ways to do so. If your child won't practice his speech homework with you, perhaps he'll agree to working with his sibling. They can make a game out of it, with each child having a turn as the teacher and student. Encourage your other kids to pretend play with your speech-disordered child—whether they're playing pirates or throwing the resident stuffed animals a tea party, such activities naturally encourage talking. I still remember the time Max told me, "Mom, I'm teaching Ari words she doesn't know." I'll admit I was initially concerned he was going to teach her how to say "stupid baby mommy," his preferred choice of curse words. But what I overheard was this:

Max: Ari, say Obi-Wan Kenobi
Ari: Obi-Wan Kenobi
Max: Say Jar Jar Binks
Ari: Jar Jar Binks
Max: Say Luke's robot hand
Ari: Luke's robot hand

Max wasn't trying to teach Ari the worst words he knew . . . he was teaching her his favorites.

Help Siblings Cope

- Give your children books to read about language challenges, as well as differences of any kind, to promote understanding and empathy. (See "Resources for Siblings.")
- Be open and honest about your child's disability and how it affects the family. Validate their feelings—whatever they may be.
- Teach your children about the communication disorder and how to best communicate with their sibling. Enlist them to help with practice sessions if they're interested, but don't force them.
- Give them the words to explain their sibling's disorder to others who may ask about it. Practice what they might say if someone says something hurtful.
- Schedule special time with all your children. They may feel neglected by all the attention your other child requires.
- Connect your kids with other siblings of children with special needs. Look for support groups online or through your therapy center or local hospital. (See the sidebar for more information.) If you can't find one, start your own.

YOUR JOB

Ari's arrival coincided with the rebirth of the advertising magazine I used to edit; it, like my new baby, was growing, from a bi-monthly to a monthly publication schedule. The three days a week I had been working for over four years wouldn't be enough to manage the increased workload. My publisher needed me a full four days a week. I wasn't happy about the increased hours, but I agreed to it because I loved the work.

My maternity leave ended right around the time we received Max's apraxia diagnosis. So with a fog in my head, a knot in my stomach, and still no idea how I was going to get Max to and from speech therapy and still meet my required hours, I returned to work. It didn't take me long to realize I was screwed.

Resources for Siblings

Books

Views from Our Shoes: Growing Up with a Brother or Sister with Special Needs, edited by Donald J. Meyer
A collection of 45 short essays from children ages four to eighteen, sharing what it's like to be the sibling of someone with a disability.

The Sibling Slam Book: What It's Really Like to Have a Brother or Sister with Special Needs, edited by Donald J. Meyer
Eighty teenagers share what it's like to have a brother or sister with special needs. Formatted like the slam books passed around schools, this one poses questions such as, "Do you like hanging out with your sib?" and "What do you tell your friends about your sib's disability?"

Hooway for Wodney Wat by Helen Lester
Wodney is a shy rat who can't pronounce his r's. Despite his speech problem, or rather, thanks to his speech problem, he's able to outsmart the new bully in class.

Sarah's Surprise by Nan Holcomb
Six-year-old Sarah is unable to talk, but with help from her therapist and a new augmentative communication device, she's able to wish her mother a happy birthday.

Charlie Who Couldn't Say His Name by Davene Fahy
Five-year-old Charlie is frustrated by his inability to correctly pronounce his name. But with help from the school speech therapist, he is able to overcome his speech difficulty.

Ruby Mae Has Something to Say by David Small
Ruby Mae is an adult with an important message of peace she'd like to deliver to the United Nations. However, she has trouble speaking and often mixes up her words. When her nephew invents a crazy hat, Ruby Mae is able to speak clearly and intelligently.

(continued on next page)

Online

The Sibling Support Project
siblingsupport.org
The goal of this national program is to promote peer support and educational programs for siblings of people with special needs. They do this through their entertaining workshops, Sibshops, as well as the Sib-Kids Listserv.

On one of my first days back I fell asleep at my desk. And when one of my regular writers quit via e-mail I burst into tears. Between adjusting to the new work schedule, dealing with Max's appointments, and awaiting the final word on his therapy treatment, I was always on the verge of tears. The fact that I was just a few months postpartum, I'm sure, didn't help. There had been a time I thought I'd actually be able to convince my boss to let me work less than the twenty-eight hours she felt the job now required. Considering I'd been behind since day two, I wouldn't have been negotiating from a position of strength. I remember looking at the stack of papers I had brought home in a vain attempt to catch up on my reading, and feared it was a position I'd lost forever.

Greater still was my fear that what I'd lost forever was a normal child. Despite everything, Max was, for the most part, a happy kid. He played with his trucks, laughed with Elmo and Blue, and enjoyed his bedtime stories just like most two-and-a-half-year-olds. But he had a very long road ahead of him, and where it was going to lead I just didn't know.

I was trying to get back into a groove—not an easy task when your sleep has been cut, your workload doubled, and the future development of your child called into question. I was supposed to be planning the March and April issues of the magazine—writing creative briefs for our cover stories, hiring freelancers to write them, making sure our regular contributors were filled in on all the changes

> ## Parent to Parent
>
> "Russell's diagnosis hasn't really affected his older brother much . . . other than at times, he's our main translator."
> > —*Pamela, mom to two-and-a-half-year-old Russell, dysphagia and sensory integration disorder (Tulsa, Oklahoma)*
>
> "When Jonathon was five he said to me, 'Karisa doesn't talk.' I told him that he was right, that she has a hard time talking and that Mrs. D. is helping her with that. His response? 'I will help her, too.' "
> > —*Mary, mom to seven-year-old Karisa, severe apraxia, sensory integration disorder, and cognitive delays, and five-and-a-half-year-old Jonathon, mild apraxia, sensory integration disorder (Louisville, Kentucky)*

taking place. Never one to have trouble managing the details or meeting deadlines, I found myself lost in thought. I was supposed to be planning an article on the best local advertising and another profiling unusual jobs in the film and video community. But I had a hard time caring about which local ads were the most creative in communicating the client's message when my own son wasn't even able to ask me for milk. And I didn't understand how I was expected to give a damn about locating an animal wrangler or special effects expert when I was still looking for a private speech therapist to teach Max how to talk.

Leaving a job I loved was hard for me; but making the decision to do so, that was easy. Max needed me and that was all there was to it. Were we nervous about the loss of income? Yes. Was I worried about keeping my career going? Of course. But these concerns paled in comparison to the ones we had for Max.

Our family certainly wasn't alone in this situation. In 2001, the federal Maternal and Child Health Care Bureau conducted a survey of children with special health-care needs. Almost 30 percent of the families interviewed reported that they needed to either cut back on work or stop working altogether as a result of their child's health-care needs.

"Initially, I quit my job," says mom Rachel. "It is impossible to expect a sitter to take a child to all the therapy appointments that are needed."

Whether you decide to stop working because of the logistics or the emotional energy that having a child with a communication problem requires, families experience this loss of income at a time when their expenses—doctor appointments, speech therapy, complementary therapies—have suddenly increased. So it's no surprise that a study out of Massachusetts General Hospital found that 40 percent of the families with children with special health-care needs they surveyed experienced a financial burden related to their child's condition.

If you'd rather not—or can't afford to—stop working, remember that your child may be eligible for speech therapy through early intervention services or the public schools. Services are free of charge and are provided during the school day, leaving you free from chauffeuring duty.

You can also:

- Talk with your boss about alternative work options such as flextime hours, moving to part-time status, telecommuting, or job sharing before making the decision to leave.
- Recruit a family member or trusted babysitter to help in getting your child to and from speech therapy.
- Find a speech therapist who will come to your home or to your child's daycare provider.

If you decide cutting back or leaving work is what's best for your family, know that there is financial assistance and affordable treatment from a variety of sources:

- Some university speech clinics offer services free of charge or on a sliding scale. The Council of Academic Programs in Communication Sciences and Disorders has a national directory at capcsd. org/cgi-bin/caplist.exe.

- Organizations such as The Knights of Columbus, Easter Seals, United Way, and Scottish Rite of Freemasonry offer financial assistance for families who need help paying for speech therapy. Contact them to see if you qualify. (For a complete list, see page 233.)
- If your child qualifies for services through early intervention or special education, she can receive therapy during the day while she's at school, free of charge.

If you do decide to leave your job, keep in touch with your boss and coworkers. Meet for lunch. Keep them posted on how your child is doing. Once you have a better handle on your child's diagnosis and treatment, and you begin to see improvement, you may no longer feel it crucial to be at home full-time. Maintaining those relationships will make it easier to go back to work—if and when you decide to do so.

"My company has been very supportive of the time I've needed to take my son to therapy," says Pamela, mom to two-and-a-half-year-old Russell. "Still, I gave my boss a video of my son for a couple of reasons. I wanted him to see what Russell has to go through just to get sentences out. And I wanted him to know that I wasn't just sleeping in late on Tuesday mornings."

Parent to Parent

"The daycare where my sons go is owned by a woman whose own son had some delays, so she was familiar with this arena. There are a couple of other kids she watches who have had issues, too. When we got an extra session of speech, she was very accommodating, and the therapist would go there to work with Daniel."

—*Denise, mom to four-year-old Daniel, speech delay*
(Huntington, New York)

The Family and Medical Leave Act

This federal law provides job protection to parents who need to take time off from work to tend to a child with a health concern and yes, that includes a speech or language disorder. Under this law, you can take an unpaid leave of absence—as brief as a few hours a week or as long as three months—with the guarantee of having a job to return to.

For parents who require regular short-term leaves of absence—which you may need to take your child to speech therapy twice a week, for example—employers have the right to make reasonable job reassignments. However, your salary and benefits must stay intact.

You are eligible for protection under the Family and Medical Leave Act if:

- You have been working in your current position for at least twelve months
- You worked no less than 1,250 hours in the last twelve months
- Your employer has at least fifty employees within seventy-five miles of their job site
- You intend to return to your job at the end of your leave

This chapter undoubtedly raised some questions about the future—the future of your child's well-being as well as your own, your marriage, your other children, and your job. It also offered up some tools for handling potential problems, and I hope you find them helpful. The next chapter addresses more immediate concerns. What you can do now—today—to encourage and improve your child's communication.

9

Home/Work: Creating a Communication-Friendly Home

Max may have been the one attending speech therapy four days a week, but he wasn't the only one developing new communication skills.

While he struggled to increase the length of his sentences, I was learning how to shorten mine. I realized, after observing his sessions for several weeks, that the SLP interacted with Max much differently than I did. I knew if I wanted to see the same improvements at home that I witnessed during therapy, I was going to have to adjust the way I talked with Max.

I knew I was guilty of using too many words with him. I would stand at the refrigerator and ask, "Max, are you thirsty? Do you want to drink some milk?" I quickly learned that simply asking him, "Milk?" was just as effective and much easier for him to process. I learned that offering him choices—"Cheese stick or apple slice?"—was far more productive than asking, "What do you want to eat?" And rather than anticipate his every want, I tried to create opportunities for Max to ask for things.

Your child's speech therapist may be the trained professional with all the letters after her name, but she needs your help in improving your child's speech or language disorder. To think that therapy, on its own, will solve your child's problem is like putting a Band-Aid on a broken arm—not too effective. Yes, the SLP is doing important work with your child; but it's likely that she only sees him in half-hour increments a few times a week. You, as the parent, spend far more time with your child. And it's time that can be spent helping him.

Key to your child's progress will be the extent to which you carry over into your home the work being done in therapy. This can be done through practice sheets or exercises the SLP gives you each week to support what is currently being taught. Even more important are the ways in which you communicate and interact with your child on a daily basis. Every interaction can become a teachable moment, as you'll see from some of the examples that follow. As you continue to observe your child's therapy, talk with the SLP and read the progress notes, you'll learn more and more how to adjust your communication to bring out the best in your child's.

ENCOURAGING COMMUNICATION

Talking to our kids is important—even at an early age. Many parents seem to naturally keep a running dialogue of what they're doing when talking to a baby. ("Jenna's in the tub getting nice and clean. Doesn't the warm water feel good? Let me see those piggy toes.") They may not realize it, but this early communication is important for your child's later language development. "When children are immersed in language, they tend to use their language earlier and more efficiently," write Roberta Michnick Golinkoff and Kathy Hirsh-Pasek in *How Babies Talk: The Magic and Mystery of Language in the First Three Years of Life.*

Whatever your child's age, regardless of where he is in his language development, there are many things you can do to encourage communication.

Respect Your Child's Struggles

Acknowledge that communication is difficult for your child ("I know sometimes it's hard for you to get the words out.") and praise

his efforts. ("I like how you used your words to tell me you're upset.")
Accept him for who he is.

Model Good Speech Behaviors

- Try not to talk too quickly.
- Use clear speech, short sentences, and simple vocabulary.
- Repeat what your child says so he knows you understand him.
- Avoid talking to your child from another room.
- Be patient and supportive. When correcting an error, be aware of your tone of voice—you don't want your child to think that you are irritated by his imperfect speech.

Get Family Support

Instruct family members and caregivers on the best way to communicate with your child. Even the children in the family who aren't struggling with speech or language will benefit from clear, thoughtful communications and no interruptions.

Make the Most of Meal Times

I realize that given today's hectic schedules filled with soccer games, committee meetings, and piano lessons, having the whole family sit down to a meal may not be a daily occurrence. When you are able to eat together, take advantage of this time to engage all the kids in conversation. Give each one a turn to talk without interruption. Ask questions about their day that require more than a one-word answer. Show your child you're interested in what he has to say.

Read to Your Child; Then, Read Some More

Listening to stories is an opportunity for your child to learn new vocabulary words and develop receptive language skills, among

Modeling 101

If you're trying to model an example of a specific speech target to a child with a speech sound disorder, there's a right and wrong way to go about doing it, according to certified practicing speech pathologist Caroline Bowen, Ph.D., of New South Wales, Australia.

Ineffective modeling
Child: That's a bid bird.
Parent: Not a bid bird. A big bird.
The child hears "bid" twice and "big" only once.

Child: That's a bid bird.
Parent: Not a bid bird. You don't say 'bid bird.' You have to remember to say 'big bird.'
The child hears "bid" three times and "big" only once. Assuming she is still listening to the explanation.

Child: He hurt his weg.
Parent: Hurt his weg? What are you supposed to say?
No speech model is provided. The child most likely feels confused and made fun of.

Child: I want the wed one.
Parent: You want the which one?
Again, no speech model is provided for the child.

Child: That's a bid bird.
Parent: It is. It is a big bird.
Here, the parent has modeled the word correctly for the child, and, for the typical language learner, it is sufficient. But a child with a speech sound disorder requires more repetitions.

Effective modeling

These examples are effective because they provide the child with multiple exposures to the correct speech sound, in proper words, and in context:

Child: I like his punny pace.
Parent: I like his funny face, too. It's a really funny face. A funny face. Do you know what that guy with the funny face is called?

Child: Det it down!
Parent: Get what down? Oh, get this down? OK. I'll get it for you. I think I can reach it. Uh-huh, I can get it.

One particular modeling technique Bowen describes is recasting. It involves repeating a word or phrase a child has said incorrectly back to her in the same words, but with the pronunciation or grammatical error corrected. Here are some examples:

Recasting for grammar
Child: I maked my bed.
Parent: I made my bed.

Recasting for speech sounds
Child: I want the lellow one.
Parent: I want the yellow one.

The suggested frequency of recasting is twelve to eighteen "recasts" within a minute for as few as three or four minutes of any given day. Here, Bowen illustrates how you can fit in up to as many as eighteen recasts in a single exchange:

Child: Him's tar talled Batmobile.
Parent: His car? (1) His car's (2) called Batmobile? That's a strange name for a car (3). Our car's (4) a Toyota. Our car's (5) not a Batmobile! You have a lot of cars (6) there! Is one of those cars (7) a Batmobile car (8)?

(continued on next page)

Child: This tar is. It he's Batmobile tar.
Parent: This car (9). Oh! This car's (10) the Batmobile car (11). Not this car (12), not this car (13), not this car (14), not this car (15). It's *this* car (16). May I play cars (17) with you? Who's driving the Bat car (18)?
Child: Me drive Bat tar . . . car.

Source: Adapted with permission from Bowen, C. (2006). Consumer slide shows for Speech-Language Pathologists to share with families, teachers and others. Retrieved September 2, 2006, from speech-language-therapy.com/ shows.html.

other things. According to Kenn Apel and Julie J. Masterson, authors of *Beyond Baby Talk: From Sounds to Sentences—A Parent's Complete Guide to Language Development,* toddlers should eventually move from reading picture books, which encourage labeling, to those that involve a sequence of events. This helps him understand more complicated sentence structures and how to relate information in a time-ordered, logical manner. Let your child hold the book and turn the pages so that she participates fully.

Create Opportunities for Communication

- Build upon something your child says. If she says, "doggie," you can respond with, "Yes, that's our doggie. Our doggie is Marnie. Marnie likes to run and chase squirrels."
- Rather than ask questions that require only a yes or no response, offer your child choices so he has to tell you what he wants. (Blue or red shorts? *Cinderella* or *Sleeping Beauty?* Hot dog or macaroni and cheese?)
- Help your child in following instructions—place your hand over hers if need be and guide her—so she links the message and the meaning. ("We're picking up the crayons.")

- When playing with toys that have many pieces (blocks, puzzles, cars), have your child request "more" before handing over the next piece.
- When coloring, have your child ask for a new color before giving her another crayon or marker.
- Whether you're pulling him in a wagon, pushing him on a swing, or playing a game of catch, stop the action every so often. Wait for him to request more.
- Teach the concept of categories by naming (either you or your child, depending on her ability) each piece of clothing as she dresses and each body part as you bathe her.

SPECIFIC STRATEGIES FOR YOUR CHILD'S DIAGNOSIS

Apraxia

- Reduce your child's frustration level by using an alternative means of communication. This isn't instead of speech therapy, but rather, something to supplement therapy in the early stages. Create themed picture boards he can point to in order to communicate his wants and help him understand your requests. For example, have a board with pictures of food to help at mealtime; another with pictures of your child's daily activities, such as getting dressed and taking a bath; another showing extended family members. Augmentative communication devices—basically, high-tech versions of the picture boards—are another option. Sign language can also be helpful in increasing spoken vocabulary, reducing frustration and differentiating words that sound the same during the early course of treatment. Depending on your child's age and abilities, you can try using American Sign Language or the more simplified Baby Signs®, which relies on simple gestures to represent things (cat, book) and concepts (all done, more) and is commonly used by many parents—not just those of kids with communication challenges. You can learn more at babysigns.com.

- Have appropriate expectations of your child. Once you know he is capable of making speech attempts, stop responding to the grunting, screaming, and pointing. Let him know you expect him to use his words, no matter how few or poorly articulated they may be. If he's standing next to the fridge and pointing, don't just hand him what he wants. Say, "Oh, would you like some milk?" When he indicates yes, say, "Tell me 'more milk.'" Model it for him one word at a time. Even a single "mmm" should be lavished with praise. It's not perfect speech you're expecting, but simply an *attempt* on his part. Once your child has improved his articulation, don't accept the approximations he used when he was younger. If you know he can clearly say "juice," don't allow him to continue requesting, "ooh." Model the correct pronunciation, and ask him to repeat it before handing over the cup.
- When reading a familiar book, leave out a word and let your child say it. ("Brown bear, brown bear what do you ___?") This also works for singing favorite songs.
- Help develop your child's functional language by working with her on important phrases such as *help me, I want, my turn,* and *more* ___.
- Reinforce any verbal attempts with praise.

Articulation

- Speak slowly and clearly. Bring toys or objects that are the topic of conversation near your mouth so your child can see how the word looks when it is being said.
- Have appropriate expectations of your child. Once you know he is able to clearly pronounce a particular word, let him know you expect him to say it properly rather than rely on old habits. If he says, "I have the *lello* crayon," you can respond with, "Yes, that's a pretty *yellow*. Let me hear you say it—*YEH-low.*"
- Encourage practice of sounds over which she has minimal control—but keep it fun. Make a game out of it, for example, by ask-

ing her to find things in the kitchen that begin with the *g* sound (garbage, grapes, glasses, garlic, etc.).

Auditory Processing

- Get his attention before talking to him. Call his name and wait for a response, or touch him on the shoulder; this will give him the cue that he needs to listen.
- Use brief instructions. Use simple language and slow, clear speech.
- Use nonverbal cues to help him understand what you're saying.
- Monitor your child's comprehension by periodically asking him questions about a book you're reading together.
- If your child misunderstands something you're telling him, repeating yourself may not be enough. Try rephrasing it.
- Reduce background noise. Turn off the TV, radio, or dishwasher when talking with your child.
- Assume that your child's failure to comply is most likely a failure to understand.

Dysarthria

- Help your child maintain good posture—for standing or sitting—as this allows for greater breath support. You may need to work with an occupational or physical therapist.
- Have your child do only one thing at a time; it may be too difficult to walk and talk.
- Be patient. Your child's language may be slow and labored, but she still wants to share her thoughts and ideas. Give her the time to get the words out and you'll be rewarded with big ideas.

Dysfluency

- Create a relaxed environment at home, and give your child opportunities to speak; set aside times when you won't be interrupted.

- Talk with your child in a relaxed, unhurried way, pausing frequently. Wait a few seconds after your child finishes speaking before you respond. According to The Stuttering Foundation of America, your own slow, relaxed speech will be far more effective than any criticism or advice such as "slow down" or "try it again."
- Reduce the number of questions you ask. She'll speak more freely if she's expressing her own ideas rather than answering an adult's questions. Rather than asking questions, try simply commenting on what she says to let her know you heard her.
- Don't finish his thoughts. Wait for him to say the intended word and listen attentively.
- Don't criticize or ask your child to repeat stuttered words until they are spoken fluently. Don't correct his speech or ask him to start over.
- Help all family members learn to take turns talking and listening. Your child will find it easier to talk when there are few interruptions and they have the listener's attention.
- Use facial expressions, eye contact, and other body language to convey that you are listening to what he is saying and not to how he is saying it.
- Set aside time each day when you can give your child your undivided attention. Let him decide how you'll spend the time and whether or not there's conversation. This quiet time can boost your child's confidence and let him know you enjoy his company.
- Talk openly about her stuttering if she brings it up.
- Convey that you accept your child just as he or she is.

Expressive/Receptive Language

- Give your child enough time to respond to you.
- Respond to a child's intended message rather than correcting her pronunciation or grammar. If she says, "That's how it doesn't go," respond, "You're right. That's not how it goes."

- Narrate what you are doing ("Mommy is making chicken soup for dinner.") and what he is doing ("You're having a nice cuddle with Lambie.")
- Play games identifying body parts. ("Show me your nose. Can you show me daddy's nose?")
- Expand upon what she says. If she says, "ball," you respond with, "yes, that's a big, green ball."
- Use repetition to reinforce language. ("Are you feeding your baby doll carrots? Does she like carrots? I like carrots. Carrots are crunchy.")

Phonological Disorder

- Speak slowly and use simple language. Be sure to clearly articulate those sound pairs (*g/d*, *c/t*) he has trouble with. ("How did it *go* today at school?" "Would you put your *cars* away please?")
- Respond to your child's intended message rather than correcting her pronunciation or grammar. If she asks for a "poon" for her cereal, respond with, "here's a spoon."
- Reduce your child's frustration level by creating themed picture boards he can point to in order to communicate his wants and help him understand your requests. For example, have a board with pictures of food to help at mealtime; another with pictures of your child's daily activities, such as getting dressed and taking a bath.
- Read books together that have a lot of rhymes. Play word games. Start an alliteration and see if he can keep it going. ("Silly Sophie sings . . . ")

Semantic-Pragmatics

- Give simple, explicit explanations. ("Put the cars in the box" rather than "clean up.")
- Avoid using sarcasm and metaphors.

- Have your child repeat what you say if you suspect he didn't understand you.
- Respond to a child's intended message rather than correcting her pronunciation or grammar. If she says, "Where my dolly is?" respond, "I don't know. Where is your dolly?"
- Take advantage of everyday routines and interactions to increase his use of different language functions. Practice greetings in the morning; have your child ask his playdate what he would like for a snack; have her request the materials she needs for an art project.
- Encourage use of effective persuasion. Ask your child how he would convince you to let him do something. Explain polite ("May I please have some ice cream?") vs. impolite ("I want ice cream now.") ways to present a request, as well as indirect ("That music is loud.") vs. direct ("Please lower the volume.")
- To develop conversation skills, be sure to comment on your child's topic of conversation before introducing a new one. Add related information. This will help your child say more about a particular subject.
- Provide visual cues such as pictures or objects to help your child tell a story in sequence.
- Encourage your child to rephrase an unclear word or sentence. If she has trouble, offer an appropriate revision by asking, "Did you mean . . . ?"
- Role-play appropriate behavior. Use his favorite action figures or her stuffed animals to demonstrate how to greet the teacher or how to share toys with a friend.
- Make use of "social stories," the short, straightforward descriptions of social situations that detail what your child might expect from a situation and what may be expected of him. They're especially helpful for teaching routines or preparing for a new experience, such as attending a wedding.
- If he has trouble responding to someone else, "give" him the words. ("Brody, if you don't want the juice box tell Mrs. Hamilton

'no thank you.' ") He may not respond because he didn't under-stand what was said or wasn't sure what kind of response to give. You could also paraphrase what was said to him in simpler lan-guage and let him respond on his own. ("Madison wants to know what you liked best about the movie.")

Voice

- Take care of your child's allergies and sinus or respiratory problems so he doesn't have to cough, sneeze, or clear his throat frequently. Reflux should also be treated to minimize its effect on the voice.
- Don't let your child talk over loud noises. Turn off the radio in the car. Turn off the dishwasher when he comes into the kitchen to talk to you.
- Help your child get in the habit of walking over to the person he wishes to speak to rather than yelling from another room in the house.
- Model a soft speaking voice; use a whistle sound to get her atten-tion from a distance.

SPEECH HOMEWORK

Your child's speech therapist will likely give you "homework" to do with your child at home. It might be a sheet of paper with pictures of a ball, bird, and bathtub if your child is working on clear articulation of the initial "b" sound. It could be a series of pictures that, when put in the right order, tells a story; this is the kind of homework to expect if your child is working on developing his sequencing and narrative skills. When Ari was having trouble with "he" and "she," and drop-ping the word "is" from simple sentences, her therapist sent home pages that featured boys and girls doing different things—walking, painting, crying, running. For each picture, I asked her "What is he (or she) doing?" If Ari answered with only the verb—"laughing"—I would prompt her by starting the sentence for her, "She . . . " Ari would get what I wanted from her and say the complete sentence: "She is laughing." To work on pronouns I would point to each picture and ask, "Who is crying? Who is riding a horse?" Ari was expected to respond with the correct pronoun: "He is. She is."

Ari was only too happy to do these exercises with me, so we would sit at the kitchen table and in just five minutes we were able to review all the exercises her SLP sent home.

Max, on the other hand, wasn't so interested in doing speech homework. Oh, he was perfectly cooperative with his therapists. But when I would sit down with him to go through the same flashcards he used with his private SLP—flashcards I paid $150 for, mind you—he didn't have much patience. I had much better luck eliciting speech attempts from him during the natural course of us playing, whether we were building block towers, coloring pictures, or role-playing as Buzz Lightyear and Batman.

The point I want to make is that, yes, it's important to carry over what's being done in therapy. Some kids are willing to sit down and go through formal exercises. Many, like Max, are not. Remember that your role here is as parent, not SLP. If regular practice makes your child angry, withdrawn, or oppositional, it's best to abandon these efforts. Your child will be working hard enough as it is, and he needs your support and encouragement far more than he does additional therapy sessions at home with mom or dad as his therapist.

That is not to say there aren't other, less intrusive, more natural—and much more fun—ways for you to help your child's speech and language development.

TOYS AS SPEECH TOOLS

You've no doubt noticed the surplus of goodies crammed into every corner of your SLP's office—silly games like What's In Ned's Head, action figures including Spiderman, Darth Vader, Strawberry Short-cake and three hundred of their closest friends, art supplies, blocks, books, puzzles, and play sets sure to please any farmer- knight-

pirate- or princess-in-training. A good therapist knows that having a good selection of toys is her surest bet to keeping kid clients happy, engaged, and productive.

So whether your child enjoys a rousing game of Uno or being up to his elbows in Play-Doh, you can easily use playtime to work on his speech and language skills.

In her book *The New Language of Toys: Teaching Communication Skills to Children with Special Needs,** Sue Schwartz says "an amazing amount of language can be pulled from even the simplest toy." And she offers these teaching tips when working with a child with a language delay:

- Focus on one toy or activity at a time to prevent your child from becoming distracted.
- Play with your child at his eye level, whether he's sitting in a high-chair or you're on the floor.
- Keep play periods brief—five to ten minutes a few times a day. As your child's attention span increases, and his communication improves, increase the length and frequency of your play times.
- Know when to stop. If he gets restless, stops paying attention, or gets frustrated to the point of melting down, it's time to call it quits.

By making use of what Schwartz calls "toy dialogs," you can help your child develop his language skills within the context of play. For example, if you and your child are stacking blocks, you can take advantage of this opportunity to teach not only the words but also the concepts of *up* and *down*: "Here's one block. Now I can put one *up* on top. See it go *up* on top? Here's another one—*up* it goes. Can we do one more? *Up-up-up-up* on top. See, we made the block go *up*."

*Source: Reprinted with permission from *The New Language of Toys: Teaching Communication Skills to Children with Special Needs*, Sue Schwartz, Woodbine House, 2004, p. 55.

When you're done building, you can ask your child, "Do you want to make the blocks fall *down*? It's fun when they all crash *down* to the ground. OK, give them a push and they'll come *down*. Aaaaaaah! They all fell *down*!"

This is just one example. There are countless ways you can combine play with speech therapy at home.

Board Games

- Before each player's turn, you must say a word from the current homework. This works for any traditional board game your child enjoys—Candyland, Hi Ho Cherry-O, Life, Monopoly.
- Each person has to think of the number of target words that matches her roll of the die. (You can model the words if necessary.)
- For nontraditional games such as Hungry Hungry Hippos or Don't Break the Ice, have your child say a word in order to earn a marble or ice block; once he has earned all the pieces, the game can be played.
- To improve your child's ability to follow directions, try Twister.
- For developing question-asking skills and deductive reasoning, play Guess Who? or Guess Where?
- Word bingo or word matching games (store bought or homemade) with rhyming words are good for developing phonemic differences.

Physical Activities

- As you take turns rolling a ball back and forth, each person has to think of a new target word and articulate it correctly.
- Go bowling (in an alley or with a toy set in your home). If he's working on articulation, have him say a target word for each pin he knocks down. If he's learning categories, pick one (farm animals, vegetables, Disney characters), and have him give you an appropriate word for each pin knocked down.

- Go on a scavenger hunt around the house for things that start with the target sound your child is working on. If it's the letter *s*, you can search for socks, stickers, sister, and sink.

Guys and Dolls

- Gather up his favorite action figures or her favorite dolls and take turns describing each one. ("She is wearing a blue dress." "He has black hair.") This is a great way to teach pronouns (*"He* is a robot. *She* is a princess.") and reinforce the smaller, grammatical parts of speech ("She *is* sitting. They *are* sleeping.") as well as articles ("I want *a* cookie." "I want *the* cookie with sprinkles.").
- For teaching concepts such as *on, in, under, next to,* and *between,* round up some dollhouse furniture. Put the dolls in different positions in relation to the furniture and ask your child, "Where's Elmo? Where's Ariel?" Prompt him with hand gestures if necessary to elicit the correct answers: *in* the tub, *under* the table, *next to* the bed, *between* the chairs.
- Invite Cinderella, King Kong, and all 101 Dalmatians to a tea party. Tell Batman, Aladdin, and Snow White it's time for school. These scenarios encourage endless conversation ("Would you like cookies with your tea?" "What would you like to do at recess?") and provide children with the appropriate language they need for everyday social situations ("May I have some sugar, please?" "Raise your hand if you know the answer.")
- Have Polly Pocket visit the library to practice using a quiet voice. Introduce her to Dora's baby brother and sister, as well as her parents, to practice using different tones and vocabulary when speaking with children and adults

TALK SHOW, OR, HOW TV CAN HELP YOUR CHILD TALK

Yes, I know. The American Academy of Pediatrics does not recommend television for children age two and younger. For those older than two, they recommend no more than one to two hours per day. I knew this back when Max was really into watching Disney movies—and not so much into talking. He was around two and a half, three years old.

Once Max was able to imitate sounds, then words, his vocabulary quickly blossomed. He could say almost anything that was asked of him. The next transition for him was initiating conversations—something he did quite a bit when we watched TV.

"Guys go boom," he'd tell me as Cruella's lackeys take a tumble in *101 Dalmatians.* "Bad guy," he said as the Huns make their appearance in *Mulan.* "Blue shark," he cried as one readies itself to pounce on Flounder and Ariel in *The Little Mermaid.* Once, Max would have just sat quietly watching. But now I got a running narrative. I didn't know who to credit more: his speech therapists or Walt Disney.

Of course that's not to say that a parent should just plant their communication-challenged child in front of the set and expect miracles. But there are ways to use television to your child's advantage. Common sense (and the AAP) suggest:

- Setting limits
- Planning your child's viewing, rather than just flipping through channels to find something
- Choosing something age-appropriate
- Watching with your child and talking about what you see

According to the National Literacy Trust, a United Kingdom nonprofit organization dedicated to literacy, there is evidence that, given the right conditions, children between two and five years of age may experience benefits—specific to language development—from quality educational television. Areas of development that might benefit include attention and comprehension, receptive vocabulary, some expressive language, letter-sound knowledge, and knowledge of narrative and storytelling. (I can certainly tell you at least one vocabulary word that Ari learned as a result of watching TV: *appro-*

priate. As in, "Ari, that show you're watching is not *appropriate* and I'm going to change the channel.")

The same study indicates that for the child to have a "positive viewing experience" certain factors need to be in place: a balance between new and familiar words, interesting material to encourage parents to watch alongside their child, use of some sophisticated language, and formats that offer possibilities for interaction and participation through songs and questions. When you think of some of the popular educational children's programming—*Sesame Street, Dora the Explorer, Blue's Clues*—they all meet this criteria.

Even the not-so-educational programs can be used to help your child. Whether your child enjoys *The Fairly Oddparents* or *Power Rangers Mystic Force*, you can take advantage of his or her interest by asking your child what has happened so far. (Develops narrative skills.) Talk about the characters and the emotions they're feeling. (Reading nonverbal cues, using appropriate social language.) Ask your child to guess how the show will end. (Reasoning and predicting skills.)

One of the most important messages I want you to take from this chapter is that your child's communication problems are not a reflection of your abilities as a parent. How early she starts talking or how easily he processes information is about as much in your control as your child's eye color, sense of humor, or natural athletic ability—it's just simply part of who your child is.

However, there are some things—such as your home environment—that are within your control. How much your child learns in this setting, it seems, is up to forces of nature—and neurobiology— we don't always understand. All you can do is provide your child with a comfortable setting where he knows he is accepted and loved. You can offer patience and maintain realistic expectations. Initiate conversations, set the pace, and practice the very communication skills you wish your child to learn.

10

School Daze: Navigating Your Way Through the Individualized Education Program

It was only a screening to see if Max warranted further evaluation through early intervention. But when the coordinator agreed to have him evaluated, I was overwhelmed with relief. Finally, the ball was in motion and we were on our way to helping Max find his voice.

She gave me a handbook explaining how the early intervention program works, and suddenly I was overwhelmed with something else. Anxiety? Dread? Fear? There was a heaviness in my chest, and I'm not sure if it was because the handbook was forty-five pages long or because the words "special education" graced the cover.

I flipped through the pages and was assaulted by words and phrases surely meant for someone else's child: mentally impaired, learning disabled, autistic. I took deep breaths, reminded myself that they give this handbook to all parents seeking services from the school and reminded myself Max's only problem is speech. Isn't it?

Ever since we received the official diagnosis of apraxia from Gail, I've felt as if I were drowning in uncertainty. Perhaps the early intervention coordinator thought she was offering a life preserver when she handed me the special education guide. But between trying to understand the logistics of getting Max "into the system" and managing my own emotions—which ranged from despair to anxiety to confusion on any given day—the handbook only served to pull me down deeper.

Needless to say, my entry into the early intervention and special education system was not smooth. There was a lot about the program I didn't know, and even more I didn't understand. Oh, I read the parent guides and talked to people. But my mind was so cluttered with questions about Max's future, I just didn't have much brainpower left for deciphering the many details of the complicated early intervention and special education systems.

If your brain is feeling bogged down, too, read on. This chapter will cover, in easy to understand language—intended for sleep-deprived, anxious parents—just about everything you need to know about getting your child free speech services.

LET'S TAKE IT FROM THE TOP

Special education doesn't refer to a specific program. It is not, as our memories of our own school days may recall, the classroom at the far end of the hall. Special education is a guarantee that students will receive an education that takes their individual needs into account.

The Individuals with Disabilities Education Act (IDEA) is the special education law in the United States. It was enacted in 1975 to ensure that children with disabilities—including speech and language—receive a free appropriate public education (FAPE). Under the IDEA, schools must provide eligible children who have a disability with an education plan that is specially designed to meet their unique needs—*at no cost to the parents.*

According to the U.S. Department of Education, for the 2003–2004 school year, more than six million students received services under IDEA. Of those, almost one and a half million received speech and language services. If your child meets certain criteria (which vary from state to state and will be covered later in this chapter), he, too, can be one of the millions of children benefiting from free speech services.

All eligible children can receive services through IDEA from birth through age twenty-two. If your child is under age three, you'll want to start with the following section on early intervention. If your child is three or older, skip ahead to Special Education. Both programs have similar processes in place for getting evaluated, qualifying for services, writing up education plans, and challenging decisions you disagree with. Where they differ is in the role of the parents and family; if your child is under three, his service plan will include how you can help your child at home, as well as different services available to assist you and the entire family. If he's older than three, the plan will focus on his education and school-related services.

EARLY INTERVENTION: BIRTH TO THREE YEARS

OK, we've already talked about IDEA. Early intervention (EI) falls under IDEA, and it supports states in providing free services for qualified young children and their families. The law requires that families and professionals work together as partners to develop a plan that identifies your child's strengths and needs and offers solutions and resources for the child, parent, and the entire family. This family-centered approach is the foundation of early intervention.

Depending on where you live, EI may go by another name. For example, in Michigan, it's known as Early On. California calls their program Early Start. In Georgia, it's Babies Can't Wait. You would find SoonerStart in Oklahoma, and First Steps in Indiana.

Adding to the confusion is that, depending on your state, the EI program may be handled by any number of organizations, including the departments of social service, mental health, public health, or education.

So, how are you supposed to know whom to call? Perhaps the easiest thing you can do is contact a school in your neighborhood.

Any school. Someone in the office will be able to direct you to the appropriate agency. You can also go online and visit the National Dissemination Center for Children with Disabilities at nichcy.org/states.htm for a state-by-state breakdown of contact information for all special education agencies and state offices.

So, How Does This Work?

Screening. You now have the name and number of the early intervention provider in your area. Call her. You'll most likely talk with a family service coordinator. Tell her your concerns. She'll ask you questions to help decide if your child requires an evaluation—this is the screening, and it's the first step in the process.

Referral. The next step is the referral. If the coordinator decides that your child should be evaluated, she'll make a referral for an evaluation. She's required to do so within two working days from your initial date of contact.

Evaluation. You and your child will meet with the evaluation team, the members of which will vary depending on your particular concerns. Of course there will be a speech therapist. But if you also have concerns about your child's behavior or fine motor skills, for example, the team may also include a child psychologist or occupational therapist. Your child's doctor can also participate—in person, by phone, or by sending a written report. This may be useful for children with complex medical problems that will have an impact on their education. There is no charge for the evaluation; the team only requires your permission. They'll look at five different areas of your child's development: physical, cognitive, communication, social/emotional, and adaptive. Depending on your state's guidelines, you may not need an evaluation if your child has already received one by another agency.

If the team determines that your child requires services, the next step will be to create an Individualized Family Service Plan (IFSP), the document that will guide you and your child through the early intervention program.

The IFSP: Putting It Down on Paper

Using information gained from the evaluation, the IFSP will detail your child's strengths and needs, your concerns, and a range of appropriate services and programs. There are specific elements, according to law, that must be included in your IFSP:

- Your child's present level of development (as determined by the evaluation)
- Your family's resources, priorities, and concerns regarding your child's development
- The expected outcomes for your child (as determined by you and the EI team)
- The criteria, procedures, and timelines to be used to determine your child's progress
- A list of the specific early intervention services that will be provided to your child and your family, as well as when, where, and how they will be provided
- How often services will be provided
- When services will begin
- How long services will be provided
- Steps to support your child's transition, at age three, to preschool or other appropriate services
- The name of the service provider responsible for implementing the IFSP and coordinating with relevant agencies

To give you a better idea of what to expect, the following chart shows some information from Ari's IFSP.

Ari's Family Service Plan

Evaluation Information Areas of Development	Family Input	Primary Findings from Evaluations and Observations
Health and Medical	No concern	(Note: Ari's IFSP was conducted close to the end of the school year so there wasn't time for a formal evaluation. We did receive one once school resumed in the fall.)
Fine and Gross Motor	No concern	
Communication	Suspected apraxia Points and squawks Few verbal attempts	
Cognitive	Does few animal sounds Uses few words on an irregular basis Self-directed behavior	
Social/Emotional	Likes others Enjoys music class	
Adaptive	Attends daycare part-time	

Strengths and Resources of Child and Family	Concerns and Needs of Child and Family
Family has been through this already. Mom is very involved with children's therapy. Both parents try to support therapy at home. Mom is home with Ari two days a week. Family is together on weekends.	Mom needs to find more one-on-one time with Ari.

Outcome	Action Service	Date	Payer
I would like to hear more verbal attempts.	Already attending private therapy Can join "Baby & Me" playgroup	 ASAP	Family Free
I want Ari to be more cooperative and to listen to suggestions.	Can join "Kindermusik" class	ASAP	Free
I want to involve both kids in activities that support Ari's speech.	Can join "Baby & Me" playgroup Contact Oakland HelpLink for additional classes and programs	ASAP ASAP	Free Free

The law indicates that the IFSP must be written within forty-five days from the date of referral. It needs to be signed by you, your coordinator, and any other service providers that may be involved in its development. If you disagree with any decisions concerning your child's services, or if you want to think about it, you can choose not to sign the IFSP and take it home for review. If you're still not happy, you'll need to negotiate for the services you believe your child requires. If an agreement can't be reached, your options are to file a formal complaint, request a hearing, or request mediation. Don't be afraid to take these steps if you feel your child is not being given what he needs.

It's advised that you bring someone with you to the IFSP planning meeting. It can be someone who can speak on behalf of your child, such as a private therapist or doctor. Or it can simply be your spouse or a friend, someone who can provide emotional support and serve as a second set of ears.

You can review and change the IFSP as often as you need to, should your child's needs change over time. Even after the initial evaluation and paperwork is taken care of, you can always ask for an assessment if you have a particular concern. Assessment differs from an evaluation in that the assessment is an ongoing process for early intervention to keep up-to-date on your child's development and progress to best determine his changing needs.

At least ninety days before your child turns three years old, your family services coordinator will write a detailed transition plan; early intervention services end when your child turns three, but your coordinator will make you aware of options for continued services and will guide you through the transition. If you feel your child still requires speech therapy, you'll most likely be directed to a new coordinator with the special education program in your area.

SPECIAL EDUCATION: THREE TO TWENTY-TWO YEARS

Whether or not your child received early intervention services—maybe you didn't have any concerns until he was four years old—he is entitled, under the law, to be evaluated for services at any age up to twenty-two years. The process is very similar to that of early intervention.

So, How Does This Work?

Like early intervention, the special education process falls under IDEA. Through what's known as Child Find, each state is required to identify and evaluate all children with disabilities. The request for evaluation can come from the parent or someone in your child's school; however, your consent for evaluation is required.

Not sure who to call to get the ball rolling? The easiest thing you can do is contact a school—any school—in your neighborhood. Someone there will be able to direct you to the appropriate office. You can also go online and visit the National Dissemination Center for Children with Disabilities at nichcy.org/states.htm for a state-by-state breakdown of contact information for all special education agencies and state offices.

OK, here's what happens after you make that first call:

Your Child Is Evaluated. An evaluation is conducted in all areas related to his suspected disability. Your child will be seen by a speech-language pathologist and, depending on any additional challenges he may have, any number of professionals including an occupational therapist, physical therapist, resource room teacher, social worker, or psychologist. The results of the evaluation will be used to determine if your child is eligible for services and to make decisions about an appropriate education for him. If you disagree with the evaluation, you have the legal right to request an Independent Educational Evaluation (IEE) that the school must pay for.

Eligibility Is Determined. If your child is found to have a disability—as defined by IDEA—he or she is eligible for special education and related services, including speech and language therapy. If your child is found to be ineligible, you can challenge this decision by asking for a hearing.

Your Child Is Found Eligible. Now the necessary personnel must convene and write an Individualized Education Program (IEP) for your child within thirty calendar days of being found eligible.

IEP Meeting Is Scheduled. In scheduling the IEP meeting, the school is required to do several things:

- Contact all participants, including the parents.
- Notify parents early enough so you can make plans to attend.
- Schedule the meeting at a time and place agreeable to you and the school.
- Tell you the purpose, time, and location of the meeting.
- Tell you who will be attending. (It could be any number of people including the speech therapist, special education teacher, and school representative. See the sidebar.)
- Inform you of your right to bring someone with you to the meeting. (It could be a friend, family member, private speech therapist, educational consultant, or anyone else who can help you advocate for your child.)

Meeting Is Held and IEP Is Written. The IEP team gathers to talk about your child's needs and write his education plan. Don't be intimidated by the number of school personnel attending or by their credentials—as the parent, you bring an expertise no one else has, and you are a vital part of the team. If your child is old enough and you feel it is appropriate, he or she may attend the meeting as well.

If you disagree with the IEP (for example, they're giving your child two half-hour speech therapy sessions a week and you want him to have three), you can try to work out an agreement. (Ask for two forty-five minute sessions per week.) If you're unable to reach a com-

---

Meet Your IEP Teammates

According to the law, certain individuals must be involved in writing your child's Individualized Education Program. However, some team members may fill more than one role if he or she is properly qualified and designated as such.

- Parents
- Student (if appropriate)
- Teachers (regular classroom and special education)
- Speech therapist (and any other provider of services, such as an occupational therapist or child psychologist)
- Someone who can interpret what the child's evaluation results mean (this could be the speech therapist)
- Someone representing the school system (such as a resource room supervisor) who is knowledgeable in special education and has the authority to commit resources
- Someone with knowledge or special expertise about your child who can lend you emotional support or help you advocate for your child (friend, relative, private therapist, professional advocate)
- Transition services representative (if your child is fourteen years old)

---

promise, you have the right to ask for mediation or file a complaint with the state education agency and request a due process hearing.

Services Are Provided. The school makes sure your child's IEP is being carried out as it was written. You are given a copy of the IEP, and your child's teachers and service providers have access to it and understand their role in following through with it.

Progress Is Measured. Your child's progress toward his annual goals is measured. You will be regularly informed of his progress, as well as whether it is enough for your child to reach his year-end goals.

IEP Is Reviewed. Your child's IEP must be reviewed at least once a year and, if necessary, it is revised. It can be reviewed more often if you or the school makes the request. Again, if you don't agree with the suggestions, IEP goals, or the placement of your child in a particular program, you can disagree. If a compromise can't be reached, you may ask for additional testing, an independent evaluation, or you can take further action challenging the school's decision. (See the sidebar.)

Your Child Is Reevaluated. At least every three years, your child must be reevaluated to determine if he continues to meet IDEA's definition of a child with a disability and what his educational needs are.

TELL ME MORE ABOUT THIS IEP

By law, an IEP must include certain information about your child and the educational program designed to meet his or her individual needs. Your child's IEP should be able to answer the following questions:

Disagree with the IEP?

Under the law, you have a right to challenge decisions about your child's eligibility, evaluation, placement, and the services the school provides. If you can't reach an agreement with the school, you have the following options:

- Mediation—Both sides (parents and school) sit down with someone who is not involved in the disagreement to try to reach an agreement.
- Due process—You and the school personnel appear before an impartial hearing officer and present your sides of the story. An officer decides how to solve the problem.
- File a complaint with the state education agency—Write a letter stating what part of IDEA you believe the school has violated. The agency must resolve the complaint within sixty calendar days.

How to Find an Advocate

If you're having trouble getting what your child needs from the school, or you're thinking about asking for a due process hearing, you may want to consult with an advocate. Some advocates are attorneys specializing in special education, educational consultants, or parents who, having already been through the system, are able to assist other parents. Here's how to find one:

Yellow Pages for Kids with Disabilities
yellowpagesforkids.com
Organized by state, this site lists hundreds of resources. In addition to advocates and attorneys, you can search for parent support groups, educational consultants, psychologists, and others who provide services to parents and children.

Parent Training and Information Centers
taalliance.org/centers/index.htm
Also organized by state, parent centers serve families of children with all disabilities and can help you find appropriate services for your child, resolve problems between you and the school, and connect you with additional community resources.

National Disability Rights Network
napas.org
This nonprofit organization offers training, technical assistance, legal support, and legislative advocacy for children—and adults—with all disabilities.

What Is My Child's Current Performance?

Evaluation results from classroom tests and assignments, individual tests given to decide eligibility for services, and observations by parents, teachers, and related service providers (including speech

Parent to Parent

"Getting the initial speech service was not difficult. Keeping her in speech therapy was. Francesca was released from receiving speech services because she was able to talk. But what she would say would not really make any sense. I had to fight to get her reinstated because of her problem with pragmatics."

—*Laura, mom to eight-year-old Francesca, apraxia, hypotonia*
(Baltimore, Maryland)

"I remember the first three years of Luke's schooling. I literally told people I loved going to IEP meetings! The people we were working with seemed so creative and energetic, and they all focused on my wonderful son. I felt like his speech therapist and teachers were colleagues of mine and we were doing our best work as a team."

—*Sharon, mom to fourteen-year-old Luke, resolved apraxia*
(Pittsburgh, Pennsylvania)

therapists) determine your child's present level of educational performance. Also included in this section is how his disability affects his involvement and progress in the general education curriculum.

What Are My Child's Annual Goals?

Annual goals, broken down into short-term objectives, are those goals that your child can reasonably accomplish in the course of a year and may address academic, social, behavioral, physical, or other educational needs. They must be measurable, relate to meeting the needs that result from the disability, and help your child be involved in the general curriculum. (For more on goals, see "Be Goal Oriented" on page 214.)

What Special Education and Related Services Will My Child Receive?

The IEP must list the special education and related services to be provided to your child including classroom or program modifications, a classroom aide, and, in this case, speech therapy services. It also includes any necessary training or professional development for school personnel who will be servicing your child.

Will My Child Participate with Children with No Apparent Disabilities?

Given the importance of developing a child's social communication skills, you can expect that your child will be placed with children who have no apparent disabilities. If for some reason this is not in the best interest of your child, the IEP will explain the extent, if any, to which your child will *not* participate with them.

Will My Child Participate in State and District-Wide Tests?

Your state and district most likely give achievement tests to children in certain grades. The IEP must spell out what modifications, if any, your child may need in order to take the test. If your child will not be participating in the tests, the IEP must explain why it's not appropriate and offer an alternative means of testing.

When and Where Will My Child Receive Services?

Your child's IEP must state when services will begin, how often they will be provided, where they will be provided, and how long they will last.

What Happens When My Child Is Approaching Graduation?

Once your child turns sixteen (or sooner, if appropriate), the IEP must include measurable post-secondary goals related to training, education, employment, and, when appropriate, independent-living skills. The transition services needed to help your child reach those goals, including your child's course of study, are also included.

When Does My Child Assume Responsibility of His Educational Rights?

Beginning at least one year before your child reaches legal age—somewhere between eighteen and twenty-one depending on your state's laws—the IEP must include a statement that the student has been told of any rights that will transfer to him. However, not all states transfer rights.

How Will My Child's Progress Be Measured?

It must be made clear how the school—or speech therapist—will measure your child's progress toward the annual goals. The IEP must also include how you will be informed of your child's progress and whether that progress is enough to allow your child to reach his annual goals. Progress reports must be given *at least* as often as they are issued to parents of children who do not receive special services.

BE GOAL ORIENTED

Your child's annual goals are those things he or she is expected to do within a twelve-month period. Short-term objectives are the steps that will help your child reach those goals and they are also written into the IEP.

Not all goals are created equally. Some are unrealistic. Others are hard to measure. Believe it or not, some IEP team members may set goals that are fairly low; goals that your child would have met without the extra help. This sometimes happens when a school is looking to eliminate specific support services.

A well-written goal should be positive and describe a skill that can be seen and measured. It also needs to indicate:

- The skill or behavior being worked on
- The manner in which it is being worked on and at what level
- The setting and conditions for meeting the goal
- The date by which the goal will be met

To give you a better idea, take a look at some of the goals from two of Max's IEPs.

This first set of goals and objectives dated December 2001 are taken from Max's very first IEP when he was two and a half years old. Because his apraxia was so severe, the therapist chose the most basic of skills to address first.

The set of goals and objectives dated December 2004 are from Max's IEP when he was five and a half years old. At this point his apraxia was considered resolved, but he still had some resulting articulation difficulties. He also needed help with his pragmatic language, and that, too, is reflected in the IEP.

What Are Well-Written Goals and Objectives?

In order to be effective, goals and objectives need to be specific, objective, quantifiable, and clear. Here are some examples:

Annual Goal
Riley will increase her semantic skills (word meaning) 75 percent as measured by SLP and teacher observations and classroom written work.

Max's Annual Goals and Short-Term Objectives, December 2001

Present level of educational performance: Max is demonstrating delays in expressive language skills.

Annual goal: For Max to increase use of core vocabulary to get basic wants/needs met.

Short-Term Objectives	Evaluation Procedures	Performance Criteria	Schedules for Evaluation
Max will imitate physical gestures.	Documentation from speech therapist	90% accuracy	Semester
Max will point, show, or give item on request.	Documentation from speech therapist	90% accuracy	Semester
Max will approximate single words for labeling and actions.	Documentation from speech therapist	90% accuracy	Semester
	Note: May also be based on teacher observations, standardized exams, rating scales, student's daily work, or other method.	Note: Can also be determined by rate (three out of four trials), production, or other criteria.	Note: Child may also be evaluated weekly, monthly, by grading period, or another predetermined schedule.

Short-Term Objectives

1. Riley will state basic personal information such as her first and last name, age, date of birth, grade, and school.
2. Riley will explain which item does not belong to a semantic category such as "Which of these does not belong? Apple, pear, shoe, banana."
3. Riley will describe objects using adjectives such as color, shape, function, composition, and texture.

Annual Goal

Jack will increase his sound discrimination through phonemic awareness to 80 percent accuracy as measured by standardized testing.

Short-Term Objectives

1. Jack will identify like sounds.
2. Jack will identify sounds and syllables contained in spoken words.
3. Jack will substitute initial sounds to create new words such as cat, fat, and mat.

Annual Goal

Zoey will use her augmentative communication device to produce a thought, comment, or idea in three out of five trials with no more than 50 percent teacher prompts or cues.

Short-Term Objectives

1. Zoey will use her device to communicate at least forty times each day.
2. Zoey will combine letter-by-letter spelling, word prediction, and preprogrammed phrases to produce a complete seven-word statement.
3. Zoey will combine letter-by-letter spelling, word prediction, and pre-programmed phrases to answer at least one "wh" question (who, what, when, where, why) in class discussions.

Max's Annual Goals and Short-Term Objectives, December 2004

Present level of educational performance: Max's articulation skills are below age level expectancies. He also has difficulty with conversational skills including turn-taking and topic maintenance.

Annual goal: To improve articulation and pragmatic language skills.

Short-Term Objectives	Evaluation Procedures	Performance Criteria	Schedules for Evaluation
Max will correctly produce the/ th/(voiceless) sound in isolation, words, sentences, and conversational speech.	Documented observation	80% accuracy	Grading period
Max will reduce his rate of speech to help increase intelligibility.	Documented observation	80% accuracy	Grading period
Max will maintain a given topic for 3–4 conversational turns and recognize and use appropriate turn-taking skills.	Documented observation	80% accuracy	Grading period

Annual Goal

Jonah will produce the phonemes k, g, and f in the initial, medial, and final positions of words and produce the phonemes m, p, b, w, t, n, and d in CVC words (words that are comprised of consonant-vowel-consonant, such as dad, map, and note) at the phrase level during structured activities 80 percent of the time.

Short-Term Objectives

1. Jonah will produce the phonemes m, p, b, w, t, n, and d in two-syllable words with 80 percent accuracy.
2. Jonah will produce the k, g, and f phonemes in isolation with 80 percent accuracy.
3. Jonah will produce the k, g, and f phonemes in the initial and final position of CVC words with 75 percent accuracy.

ELIGIBILITY EXPLAINED

Defining which children are eligible for speech and language services has been a challenge for the state education offices charged with this responsibility—not to mention the parents trying to understand a very complicated system.

The Individuals with Disabilities Education Act specifies that a child have an established condition that has a high probability of resulting in a developmental delay, or that a delay is present in one or more areas of development—cognitive, physical, communicative, social and emotional, or adaptive. However, each state is free to determine the amount of delay a child must experience in order to qualify for services. The states also have the discretion to select appropriate diagnostic tools to measure the extent of a child's delay (quantitative criteria) or to rely exclusively on the informed opinion of professionals (qualitative criteria).

Quantitative criteria are that which can be measured. For example, if a child is twenty-four months old but developmentally behaves as an eighteen-month-old, his delay would be measured at six months, or 25 percent. Qualitative criteria are that which can be observed, such as comparing the language skills of a two-year-old with that of her peers.

In order for your child to be eligible for speech therapy, he or she needs to be delayed by a certain amount. Common measurements of level of delay in many states are:

- 25 percent delay or two standard deviations below the mean in one or more developmental areas
- 20 percent delay or 1.5 standard deviations below the mean in two or more areas

A standard deviation is one way of measuring variation on standardized tests. For example, if the mean (average score) of a particular speech test were 100, and the standard deviation was 15, then a score of 85 would be considered one standard deviation below the mean. A child who scores between 85 and 115—one standard deviation from the mean of 100—would be considered to have average speech or language abilities. But if the child scored 70—two standard deviations below the mean—he would be considered below average for that particular ability being tested and likely in need of therapy.

Despite these common measurements, there is still some variability between the states. So much so, that a child who meets the criteria in one state, can be deemed ineligible in another. For example, if you live in New Jersey, your child's speech would need to be delayed by 33 percent in order to receive services. (However, a child with a 25 percent delay could also receive services—if she had another 25 percent delay in another developmental area, such as physical or cognitive.) Arizona requires a 50 percent delay in one or more areas of development. Which means the kid in Trenton will get the help he needs, but his peer in Tucson won't.

If your child is found to be ineligible, the school must tell you this—in writing—and explain why. Under the rules of IDEA, you must be given information about what you can do if you disagree with the decision.

TIPS FOR SURVIVING THE IEP PROCESS

Getting the school to give you what you want for your child requires some subtle marketing and selling strategies, according to Peter Wright, a special education attorney who provides advocacy training for parents (as well as everything you need to know about special education law on his website wrightslaw.com).

The secret to a successful IEP meeting? "Understand that the person across the table from you is responding to pressures from higher ups in the bureaucratic structure as well as economic pressures," says Wright. "Deciding what services your child receives is an economic issue rather than a personal battle. Don't get swept up in the emotions."

Some speech therapists are disheartened to hear Wright's advice. "I've never been pressured by my special education director as to how many days a week I could see kids," says Allison, a speech therapist who works for the public schools in southeastern Michigan. While she admits that her district is having trouble hiring additional speech therapists, and that her own caseload has exceeded the number of students she's permitted to have by law, it hasn't affected her ability to service her students. "I've always figured out a way to do it," she says. "I've never been in a meeting with a parent who felt we weren't seeing the child often enough. It just wouldn't be an issue. I couldn't do this job if I wasn't really helping the kids."

Still, it's important for parents to understand the law. And in many cases, it's the parents who are more knowledgeable about special education law than the educators themselves. But challenging them by telling them they are incorrect and pulling out a copy of IDEA won't help your case. Instead, it puts the IEP team on the defensive—which doesn't help you.

Wright encourages parents to instead ask questions. For example, if you're only being offered two days a week of speech therapy—and your private therapist has strongly recommended four days a week—rather than debate with the IEP team, ask them, "Why do you think your proposal of having less speech therapy is better?" It's likely they don't know themselves. So in their efforts to find that information, their needs align with yours. "The situation doesn't become polarized," says Wright.

Now that you've got your key strategy, here are additional tips to keep in mind for a successful IEP meeting:

- Before the meeting, review your child's information, including any evaluations you may have had privately as well as your own notes. If you feel the current evaluations don't present a complete picture, ask for the meeting to be postponed until more information can be obtained.
- If you have a private speech therapist or your child sees a psychologist, talk with them to get ideas of what should be included in your child's IEP.
- Bring anything with you that will help give the IEP team a better idea of your specific concerns for your child: medical records, private speech testing, samples of your child's schoolwork, audio or videotape clips.
- Be familiar with the different programs, classes, and services available to your child. Talk to other parents to find out what was offered to other students. You can't ask for particular services if you don't know they exist.
- Know your rights. Review IDEA regulations and take a copy with you to the meeting in case you need it. Understand how the IEP process works.
- Anticipate any areas where you and the school might disagree, and think about how you want to handle this. Write down any information to support your position. Bring records. Think of

alternatives to offer if the school won't accept your first suggestion. Know your bottom line.

- Plan to bring someone along to the meeting. IEPs can be emotionally charged, overwhelming, and very confusing. It helps to have someone along for moral support who can serve as an extra pair of ears and who can ask your questions should your emotions get the better of you. If you're bringing an advocate, make sure she knows your concerns before the meeting.

- Plan to bring a tape recorder. You may not remember everything that is said during the meeting, especially if things get heated. But if you're concerned that the IEP team will view this as antagonistic, pass it off under the guise of your "faulty memory." If they still resist, remind them that it's your legal right to use a recorder.

- Don't be shy about speaking up for your child's needs, even if there are a lot of people in the meeting. Don't be afraid to ask questions. Educate yourself about your child's diagnosis. Consider bringing information sheets for the entire IEP team.

- Try to maintain a good working relationship with the school and the IEP team. You're going to have to make decisions with them about your child for several years. Try to work out any disagreements with the team before taking other action. That said . . .

- Don't be afraid to take the necessary steps to challenge the IEP if you feel your child is not getting what she needs.

- Don't sign the IEP during the meeting—even if you agree with it. Take it home and review it at your own pace. Share it with your spouse, your child's private speech therapist, doctor, or anyone else who can help you evaluate it. Show it to a special education attorney or advocate if you have concerns.

SET UP YOUR CHILD FOR SUCCESS

There are things you can do to help your child in school beyond ensuring he has a well-written IEP:

- Invite a classmate over for a playdate. If your child feels too shy to talk in class, this will provide him with an opportunity to play one-on-one in a comfortable environment, and in turn, help form a connection that carries over into the classroom.

- Talk with your child's teacher about how you might volunteer in the classroom. Volunteering lets you see how your child interacts with others and how things work in the school. You'll also be able to determine if your child's IEP is being upheld.

- Explain to your child's teacher how his communication challenges may affect him in the classroom. Brainstorm with the SLP in advance to provide the teacher with strategies she can use to help your child and bring out his best. If he uses an augmentative device, explain how it works. Depending on the severity of your child's problem—and your child's desires—you might consider talking to the class about it. Tell them the name of your child's disorder and explain, in child-friendly terms, how it affects him. ("Noah's brain has trouble making his mouth work." "Darcy uses a special computer to talk for her.")

- Maintain regular communication with the teacher about your child's performance and any challenges he may be having. Ask her to maintain communication with the SLP.

Remember my initial fear when I was first handed a special education handbook? I found that the more I learned about Max's diagnosis and the better I understood what kind of therapy he needed, the less I was intimidated by special education. (The process, as

Parent to Parent

"It behooves parents to educate themselves as you are your child's best advocate. You should not abdicate that role to the so-called 'experts.'"
—*Dee, mom to ten-year-old Adam, severe verbal apraxia*
(Madison, Wisconsin)

well as the words.) In fact, years after fearing the label for my son, I was practically begging for it for my daughter. Ari's school SLP was releasing her from speech services as she was entering kindergarten and I felt she still needed help. "I don't want her to start kindergarten and have a special education label attached," the therapist said, much to my surprise. All I could think was—who cares about the label? That label means she'll get the services she needs.

Don't let the label, or a confusing system, stop you from getting your child the speech services he needs—and is entitled to. Use this chapter as your guide. Talk to other parents. Find an advocate who can help you get started. And remember, there are many people in the school system who can help your child. But the most important one is you.

The "All About Me" Book: How to Share Information About Your Child with New People

Sharon Gretz admits she was terrified when her son, Luke, diagnosed with apraxia, was ready to transition from preschool into the elementary school system. The preschool staff and his private speech language pathologist had a nice team approach in place and her son was thriving. His ability to communicate with other children and the adults at school had changed enormously. He was happy and well-adjusted. And now, he had to start over.

Sharon created the "All About Me" book because she was "scared to death" that Luke was starting kindergarten and she wouldn't be able to observe him as she had when he was in preschool. "I had a strong desire to insure that the people who were working with my son not only understood his problems, but also had the opportunity to see the wonderful little boy there," she says.

She created a questionnaire that she distributed to everyone who knew and cared about her son, including relatives, friends, teachers, and

(continued on next page)

therapists. The questions were modified versions from a planning tool called the McGill Action Planning Systems (MAPS), which is a particular method of creating an action plan for students with disabilities:

- Who is my child? (Describe special attributes and qualities. Use descriptive terms. What are the things that make him uniquely him?)
- What are his special talents and abilities?
- What are his most pressing needs at this time?
- What kinds of things are guaranteed to motivate, engage, and enthrall him?
- What kinds of things are guaranteed to cause him upset, anxiety, and concern?
- If I could tell my child's new team at school one very important thing about him, what would it be?

Everyone turned in their questionnaires to Sharon and she compiled them into an attractive booklet that listed the questions and answers. She made sure responses were not duplicated and that similar responses were grouped together. She made copies of the "All About Me" book and distributed them at her first meeting with the new school.

In the end, many people who worked with Luke during his kindergarten year, and over the next several years, told Sharon that the "All About Me" book was the most accurate and helpful piece of "paperwork" that they had received. (And given that Luke was "in the system," he certainly had a ton of paperwork that followed him.)

"The idea of 'All About Me' was to capture some of the wisdom of the people who knew and loved my son and to help the new team of professionals see him as a whole child, not just a child with special needs," says Sharon.

Source: Adapted with permission from Sharon Gretz, founder of Apraxia-KIDS © (apraxia-kids.org), a program of The Childhood Apraxia of Speech Association of North America (CASANA).

11

Are You Covered? Cutting Through the Red Tape of Insurance

Nine hundred dollars worth of insurance checks have just arrived in the mail and I can't stop crying.

It's not the financial relief that has me feeling emotional; it's the validation these checks represent.

Our previous insurance company rejected our claims for Max's speech therapy on the grounds that while they did cover speech therapy, they didn't cover treatment for developmental disorders. I went several rounds with them providing them with a wealth of information explaining how apraxia was not a developmental disorder, but rather, neurological in nature. I wrote letters. I sent copies of Max's evaluation and progress reports. Max's speech therapist talked with their "medical expert," but it was to no avail. They refused to pay.

Well, I refused to accept no for an answer. I contacted the state office that handles such matters and requested an external review. I knew I was right in expecting coverage, and I hoped the state would prove a more objective reviewer of the information than my insurance company had.

It took many months, but eventually, the state overturned all the rejected claims. Our insurance company had to pay the thousands of dollars we were due, and I couldn't have felt more victorious.

It was that sense of validation I felt when I received reimbursement from our new insurance company—without having to fight them for it. The financial relief was the least of it. I think what I felt was emotional relief; that someone finally acknowledged and understood the seriousness of Max's condition. Those three checks—just the first of many we were to receive—validated all the sacrifices we had made to get Max the help he desperately needed. I had quit a job I loved. I was constantly running to therapy appointments. And Max was working hard just so he could do what the rest of the world takes for granted: speak. By turning down our claims, our first insurer minimized the seriousness of Max's disorder and dismissed how it impacted all our lives. When our new insurance provider paid up right away, I felt victorious, yes, but even more so, I felt understood.

It can be stressful enough just trying to make sense of our children's problems and finding them the right help. The last thing most of us have the time or energy for is fighting with our insurance companies. This is made all the more apparent by one study of state external review programs that found that the 902 cases New York's program handled one year was the largest number of any state. But this translated to less than eleven cases per 100,000 insured lives in that state.

Does this mean New Yorkers are more satisfied with their insurance plans than the rest of the country? Hardly. It means that most people choose not to pursue a rejected health insurance claim. The process—assuming policyholders are even aware that such an appeal process exists—is complicated and time-consuming and most people, when it comes to paying a medical bill, will choose to finance it themselves rather than fight. Even those people who choose to challenge their health plan denials won't necessarily exhaust their health plan's internal process, let alone reach the point where they request an external review from the state. And the insurance companies are counting on that.

"Insurance companies' business models are based on the assumption that not everyone who has a right to appeal will, in fact, appeal," says Barry D. Liss, an attorney in Warren, New Jersey, specializing in health-care issues and insurance claims denials. "If everyone did, their costs would go up."

I know this whole process can leave you feeling overwhelmed and exhausted—I certainly was back when Max was first diagnosed. And by the time I had a handle on things, I was back to feeling overwhelmed and exhausted by Ari's diagnosis. But I urge you to fight for what is yours. Coverage for speech and language disorders can be tricky. And each policy has its own set of rules. But the more informed you are, the better prepared you'll be to plan an organized, compelling, and hopefully, effective case for getting the coverage your child needs.

UNDERSTAND YOUR POLICY

Start with the basics. What does your policy cover? Until now, you may not have had a reason to give your policy a close look and it may be hidden away in your basement in a file cabinet you've long forgotten about. So if you can't find it, your employer or your insurance company can provide you with another copy.

Once you've got your explanation of benefits, find the section on speech and language therapy, which may also be included under rehabilitation services, physical and occupational therapy, other medically necessary services, or therapies. You'll also want to check the "exclusions to coverage" section, also referred to as "charges covered with special limitations" and see if there's any mention of speech therapy.

If You're Covered

If your policy includes speech and language therapy, find out:

- **Are both the initial evaluation and ongoing therapy covered?** You may find the initial evaluation is covered, only to be surprised later on when your claims for therapy are denied.

- **Is therapy covered for my child's particular diagnosis?** Some policies fail to explicitly state what conditions are excluded from coverage. Your benefits handbook may indicate that speech therapy is a covered service only to later find your claims rejected based on your child's particular diagnosis. Find out from your speech therapist which diagnostic code she plans to use and ask your insurance company if they cover that specific code.

- **Is there a maximum number of therapy visits per year that will be reimbursed?** If this is the case, is it possible to get coverage for additional visits if the SLP recommends this? Also ask if coverage for speech therapy visits are combined with occupational and physical therapy visits.

- **What is the deductible or co-pay?** The deductible is the amount of money you must pay out-of-pocket before the benefits of the policy can apply. So although your plan may cover speech therapy, you are still required to meet your deductible, which could be anywhere from hundreds to thousands of dollars depending upon your particular coverage. Even after you've met the deductible, you are likely to have a co-pay for each speech session, the amount of which will again depend on your insurance plan.

- **Do I have to choose an SLP from a network of approved providers?** Some insurance plans will only provide coverage if you see a professional who's part of their network. Others may allow for service providers who are either in or out of the network, but reimburse a higher amount for in-network SLPs. Others give you free reign. You'll want to know what your options are if you're looking to keep your costs down.

- **Is prior authorization required?** Some insurance companies may require prior approval or a doctor's prescription before any services are rendered. Depending on your individual policy, this may be referred to as pre-authorization, pre-certification or pre-determination. If your pediatrician referred you for the speech evaluation, submit the referral to the insurance company. If you self-referred or were referred by a teacher or friend, you can always ask your doctor to write the letter now. Be aware that if your insurer doesn't receive it before your child is seen for the evaluation, they may refuse to pay for it.

If You're Not Covered

If your policy doesn't cover speech therapy, or has limited coverage that precludes any services for your child, there are several things you can do.

- **See if your employer offers another plan that provides coverage.** Switch during the next open enrollment.
- **Send a letter to your employer requesting better coverage.** Employers have the greatest influence in obtaining better insurance coverage as they negotiate the contracts with the insurance companies. Your employer will have no idea of the need for speech therapy coverage unless you inform them that you were denied. Group insurance coverage for speech and language evaluations and therapy is a relatively inexpensive rider for most companies to add to their existing policies. Contact the American Speech-Language-Hearing Association (asha.org or 800-638-8255) and request an Employer Insurance Packet to help you make your case.
- **Have your child evaluated by early intervention or special education services.** As discussed in earlier chapters, the public schools offer free speech therapy services to those children who meet certain criteria. If your child qualifies, push for as much service as you can get. If she doesn't qualify, ask why not. Request copies of your child's evaluations and test scores, as well as an explanation of your state's criteria for eligibility. Find a parent advocate who can help you make an argument for your child to receive services.
- **Contact university speech clinics about sliding scale or no-fee services.** Many universities with communication-disorder programs offer speech services through an affiliated clinic. Because

it serves as an academic facility, some clinics offer services free of charge or on a sliding scale. The Council of Academic Programs in Communication Sciences and Disorders has a national directory at capcsd.org/cgi-bin/caplist.exe.

- **Set up a flexible spending account.** Depending on your employer, you may be able to deduct pre-tax dollars for health-care costs. How does it work? First, you choose the amount of money you want set aside for medical costs. The money is usually taken out through regular, equal payroll deductions—on a pre-tax basis. And you can use it to help with your co-pays or for your child's speech treatment. But be sure to keep track of your spending—if you don't use all the money in your account by the end of your company's benefit year, it gets forfeited.

- **Apply for Medicaid.** The Medicaid program allows for direct reimbursement to speech pathologists. Guidelines vary from state to state; for more information, visit cms.hhs.gov.

- **Find organizations offering financial assistance.** ASHA lists many organizations that provide funding for children in need of speech and language therapy. (See the facing sidebar.) Guidelines for eligibility vary, so you will have to contact each one to learn more about their programs. It's possible your private speech therapist may be familiar with additional options, so don't hesitate to ask.

SUBMITTING A CLAIM

Some speech therapists will file health claims for you, but in most cases you'll have to handle the paperwork yourself. Find out if your insurance requires you to submit within a certain number of days from the date of service. You don't want to be denied coverage because you were late sending in the paperwork.

If this is the first time you're submitting, send any related documentation such as your physician referral, initial evaluation, or treatment plan. Take note of the diagnostic code your SLP is using (more

Financial Assistance for Speech Therapy	
BPO Elks of the USA elks.org	*Pilot International* pilotinternational.org
Civitan International civitan.org	*RESNA Technical Assistance Project* resna.org/taproject
Easter Seals easterseals.com	*Rotary International* rotary.org
Government Benefits GovBenefits.gov	*Ruritan National, Inc.* ruritan.org
Kiwanis International kiwanis.org	*Scottish Rite of Freemasonry* scottishrite.org
Knights of Columbus kofc.org	*Sertoma* sertoma.org
Lions Club International lionsclubs.org	*United HealthCare Children's Foundation, Inc.* uhccf.org
March of Dimes marchofdimes.com	*United Way* unitedway.org

on this on page 238), and make sure it isn't one that's likely to be denied. Be sure to keep copies of everything you send! Paperwork gets lost and you may need to resubmit. Keep records, including the name of the person you are submitting to as well as the date.

If Your Claim Is Denied

An explanation for any denial should be included in the paperwork you receive, but if it isn't, or it doesn't make sense to you, call your insurance company and ask. Find out which diagnostic codes they'll pay and which ones they won't. If you don't already have it, ask for a copy of your plan's policy for speech therapy services as well as an explanation for the denial in writing. Ask what information is required in order for your claim to be approved. You may be missing a seemingly insignificant piece of information, but understand that insurance companies will do what they can to reject your claim. You can make it harder for them by giving them all the information they request. Keep a record of who you talk with, when you talk with them, and what was said. Trust me—you won't remember this a month from now.

In addition to getting an explanation for the denial in writing, you'll also want to ask for:

- A statement identifying the treatment exclusion in your policy
- The name, title, medical license number, and licensing state of the person making the denial decision
- Instructions for filing an internal appeal, including whether it has to be in writing, any time limits for appealing, and the name and phone number of a contact person
- Instructions for filing an external review should your internal review yield another denial
- Contact your employer's Benefits Coordinator. Provide him with documentation of your conversations with the insurance representative as well as copies of all correspondence. Ask him to contact the insurance company on your behalf.
- Appeal the denial. Don't think a denial from your insurance company is the final word. According to a 1999 Kaiser Family Foundation study, 42 percent of doctors said that their most recent treatment denial was ultimately resolved in the patient's favor.

Every insurance company has their own process to follow for an internal appeal, that is, an appeal to the insurer itself, and the first step in what can be a long process. (An external appeal is to your state department of insurance or other governing body.) Call yours and find out what steps you have to take. You may only have a limited

Parent to Parent

"We were rejected by several insurers on the basis that there was no medical necessity and that apraxia was a developmental delay. I fought the denial and won both times that I appealed. It took lots of time, letters, and phone calls . . . I'm sure the fact that I'm a lawyer helped."

—*Dee, mom to ten-year-old Adam, severe apraxia (Madison, Wisconsin)*

"We have not collected any insurance coverage because our claims have been rejected. We have paid for all of our private speech services. It's so costly. We could have paid for private school tuition for the same cost."

—*Gerilyn, mom to seven-year-old Ryan, mixed expressive/receptive language disorder, learning disability, and six-year-old Julianne, global delay, learning disability, ADHD (Briarcliff Manor, New York)*

time from the date of therapy to start your appeal, so don't wait too long to get things rolling.

You'll need to write a letter that includes:

1. Your child's name and diagnosis
2. How the diagnosis affects your child and the family
3. The progress your child has made as a result of speech therapy
4. The prognosis for your child without the speech therapy
5. A list of the information you are enclosing, such as a physician's letter of medical necessity, letter from your speech therapist, evaluations, treatment plans, progress reports, any additional information that explains your child's diagnosis

Talk with your child's doctor first, but consider writing the letter of medical necessity yourself. Although doctors most certainly support our fight for coverage, they're busy people who may not have the necessary time to put into writing an effective letter. And, as they

---

Letter of Medical Necessity

Whether your physician writes one himself, or you write it for him, the American Speech-Language-Hearing Association recommends these important steps:

- **Educate your health plan about the nature of your child's communication disorder and relate the description to coverage language from your policy.** For example: The term apraxia of speech describes a neurologically based speech disorder that interferes with a child's ability to initiate and sequence motor movements for speech. The child has limited control of speech muscles. It is an oral-motor speech disorder characterized by the loss of ability to consistently position the articulators for speech. Unintelligible speech is the result.

- **Indicate that speech pathology treatment is medically necessary.** Describe your child's disorder as a medical condition consistent with the definition of disease and illness; it is a disorder of body function.

- **Describe the treatment plan and expected results.** For example: Children with verbal apraxia respond best to motor treatment that is focused on the control of speech movements. Carefully structured treatment programs that combine muscle movement, speech sound production, and sometimes work on grammar and expressive language skills seem to get the best results. Intensive therapy should begin as soon as the child is diagnosed and should be consistent and frequent. Without professional treatment, children with verbal apraxia will not develop normal speech. With treatment, prognosis is good.

---

are not experts on speech and language disorders, you may very well know more about your child's disorder than his doctor. Offer to write a draft the doctor can amend as needed and sign.

You'll want to send everything together in one envelope, preferably by certified mail so you will be notified when they receive it. Follow up about two weeks after sending the packet to check on the status. Don't be surprised if the process takes longer than you're initially told.

COMMON REASONS FOR INSURANCE DENIALS

Narrow Definition of "Medical Necessity"

Many pediatric speech and language disorders are caused by neurological impairments in which the exact cause can't always be explained. Without this "medical" cause, insurance plans may claim that therapy isn't medically necessary.

But here's what you have to keep in mind: the only people qualified to determine if therapy is medically necessary is your child's doctor or speech therapist—not the number cruncher at your insurance company. If your claim is turned down because of lack of medical necessity, it may simply mean that you haven't submitted sufficient information for your insurance provider to find evidence of medical necessity. Ask what additional information is needed. It may be as simple as using a different diagnostic code. Or you may need to provide more information about your child's disorder.

No Coverage for Developmental Disorders

The word "developmental" means different things to speech pathologists than it does to insurance claims officers. If "developmental" is part of your child's speech diagnosis, it's simply being used to distinguish the condition from that of an adult. However, a developmental condition is also one in which the child will catch up on his own, without therapy. Sometimes a developmental or speech delay is simply that—the child will reach his milestones, just a little bit later than his peers. Many children aren't given a speech diagnosis,

Decoding Diagnostic Codes

Take a look at your billing statement from your child's speech therapist. Or from any of your own doctors for that matter. You'll find a five digit diagnostic code that, until now, you may not have paid much attention to. That's about to change. Because the difference between 315.40 and 315.31 is far greater than just .09—it could mean the difference between getting your insurance company to pay and having to foot the bill yourself. The codes below are taken from the International Classification of Diseases (ICD) and are used by all medical professionals.

Most of the codes in the 315 range are classified by the insurance companies as delays in development. For example:

Developmental speech and language disorder	315.50
Developmental language disorder	315.31
Developmental articulation disorder	315.39
Unspecified delay in development	315.9
Receptive language disorder (mixed)	315.32

Since insurance companies make it difficult to get reimbursed for what they consider a developmental disorder, it's best to avoid using these codes—if you can. Ask your SLP if there are any other codes she can honestly use instead.

In general, diagnostic codes in the 700 range are more likely to be reimbursed. Here are some that might be relevant to your child's condition:

Aphasia (loss of ability to speak or understand speech)	784.30
Other	784.69

      Agnosia (loss of ability to recognize objects, persons, sounds, shapes, or smells)

      Agraphia (loss of ability to write)

      Apraxia

Dysarthria	784.50
Dysphagia (difficulty swallowing)	787.2
Voice disturbance, unspecified	784.40
Aphonia (loss of voice)	784.41
Other	784.49

> *Changes in voice*
>
> *Dysphonia (impairment of the voice or difficulty speaking)*
>
> *Hoarseness*
>
> *Hypernasality or hyponasality*

Other speech disturbance	784.5

> *Dysarthria*
>
> *Dysphasia (language impairment usually due to brain damage)*
>
> *Slurred speech*

If your child has another condition that is related to her speech and language difficulties, ask whether the SLP can use that code in place of the developmental codes.

For problems related to complications of the perinatal and neonatal period:

Periventricular leukomalacia (damage to the white matter of the brain)	779.7
Fetal and neonatal hemorrhage	772.1

For problems related to traumatic brain injury:

Intracranial injury	850.0
Head injury, unspecified	959.01

For genetic conditions associated with speech and language difficulties:

Spina bifida	741
Other congenital anomalies of nervous system	742

(continued on next page)

Decoding Diagnostic Codes *(continued)*	
Cleft palate and cleft lip	749
Chromosomal anomalies	758
Down syndrome	758.0
Klinefelter syndrome	758.7
Fragile X syndrome	759.83

but instead are labeled speech delayed. (These same children if "delayed" long enough, will eventually be deemed "disordered" and stand a better chance of insurance coverage.)

Even if your SLP is only identifying your child as "delayed," ask that she not use that word when writing a letter on your child's behalf. Find out what diagnostic code she plans to use—if it's one with developmental as part of the name, see if there's another one she can use.

No Rehabilitative Care for Children

Most plans will have some coverage of rehabilitative services—those services and therapies that help people regain skills they previously had, often prior to an illness or injury, such as speech therapy for someone who has suffered a stroke. But some policies will argue that the same speech therapy is not covered for a child because it is not rehabilitative, that is, the child didn't develop speech and lose his ability—he just never developed this skill in the first place (unless you could demonstrate that your child had speech and lost it, which happens with some disorders, including autism). This kind of exclusion doesn't allow for the needs of infants and young children.

"Children are developing by definition," says attorney Liss. "Every single service provided to a child is to allow them to achieve abilities they didn't previously have." You can also argue that your policy doesn't state that rehabilitative services for children are restricted.

No Coverage for Particular Disorders

If your member handbook doesn't explicitly state that a particular disorder is excluded from coverage you can appeal the rejection based on the vague phrasing of the contract. Some policies specifically identify articulation disorders and stuttering as two diagnoses not covered because they believe—incorrectly—that they are developmental in nature.

Articulation Disorder. If your child has another speech condition in addition to an articulation disorder, try resubmitting with the other diagnosis as the primary diagnosis code. Or take a page from a letter the American Speech-Language-Hearing Association wrote when advocating on behalf of a child whose speech therapy benefit was denied on the basis that articulation disorders were not covered:

"Excluding articulation disorders was noted to be perplexing because articulation disorders refer to many types of speech impairments that otherwise would be covered under the policy, such as cleft palate related speech impairments and dysarthria. ASHA observed the policy language was akin to saying it provided treatment for broken bones, except for breaks of the arm or leg."

Stuttering. Some health insurance companies will cover speech when it is rehabilitative or restorative but may deny a claim for stuttering if it's believed to be a chronic speech disability. You can argue your case by providing information about the neurological basis of stuttering, such as this tidbit from an article in *Neurology* that ran in 2001: "Researchers who studied adults with persistent stuttering found that these individuals had anatomical irregularities in the areas of the brain that control language and speech." Or borrow this argument from a sample letter in ASHA's *Appealing Health Plan Denials*: "Stuttering is an illness as it has been classified and given a diagnostic code in the *International Classification of Diseases*, 9th revision. According to *Stedman's Medical Dictionary*, 24th edition, illness is defined as 'disease,' which is further defined as a 'disorder of body functions,' and is a condition marked by deviation from the normal healthy state. Healthy means free from disease or dysfunction. The stutterer is not free from dysfunction, as evidenced by the lack of normal speech function."

No Coverage for Educational Services for Which the Public Schools Are Responsible

Yes, the public schools are responsible for providing speech therapy services to those in need—but this doesn't always happen. Not all children who need help qualify for services. And not all those who do qualify get what they need owing to overloaded caseloads or inexperienced therapists.

But none of that matters.

Whether or not your child receives speech therapy through school should be irrelevant to your insurance company. The public schools are not medical providers; they are responsible for providing a proper education for all children as covered under IDEA. And your insurance provider is responsible for providing coverage of medical needs as specified in your plan.

You can also mention that speech-language pathology services are formally recognized as health-care services by the Joint Commission on Accreditation of Healthcare Organizations, Medicare, Medicaid, and the Health Insurance Association of America.

If they ask for a copy of your IEP, be sure to specify how the school therapy differs from private therapy—you'll need a reason to warrant the private therapy. For example, the school provides group therapy and the private therapist does one-on-one.

For more information—and valid arguments you can use to make your case—visit speechville.com or pick up a copy of *Appealing Health Plan Denials*, available through the American Speech-Language-Hearing Association.

The Ideal Health Plan

- Provides benefits for all necessary speech and language services without excluding specific kinds of problems
- Pays 100 percent of allowable charges
- Pays for at least a significant portion of needed services
- Doesn't impose a pre-set limit on the number of reimbursable therapy sessions
- Doesn't impose a yearly or lifetime limit on benefits
- Provides access to a sufficient number of local speech pathologists

Source: American Speech-Language-Hearing Association (asha.org)

FILING AN EXTERNAL APPEAL

My insurance company had denied payment on Max's therapy twice. I followed all their internal procedures, submitted all the paperwork, and had my expert talk to their so-called expert. Still, they refused to pay. I could let it go—as insurance companies expect policyholders to do, and the majority do walk away from the fight—or I could take it to the next level and file an external appeal.

External appeals are filed with your state's department of insurance or other designated office. In Michigan, it's the Office of Financial and Insurance Services; in Florida, it's the Subscriber Assistance Program. However, not all states have a designated office, and if you live in such a state, you can request an independent review through your insurance company. Find out who to contact by asking your insurance company or by contacting these resources:

National Association of Insurance Commissioners
naic.org/state_web_map.htm
This site will link you directly to your state's department of
   insurance website.

Consumer Guide to Handling Disputes with Your Employer or Private Health Plan
consumersunion.org/health/hmo-review
This site details the necessary steps for filing an external appeal.

When you file an appeal you are basically asking the government to reconsider your health plan's denial of coverage. This external review, unlike your internal reviews conducted by your insurer, is conducted by individuals not affiliated with your health plan—so you can hope to receive a more objective response.

What to Expect

Your state office won't review your case until you've exhausted your options with your insurance company's process. So don't jump the gun and file with the state too early—you'll only be wasting your time.

There is some variation in procedures from state to state, but for the most part, your state office will determine if your request is eligible for an external review before sending it through to a reviewer.

Most states require that the issue at stake involve "medical necessity." Many states explicitly exclude disputes over coverage issues such as whether you can use a nonnetwork provider because no qualified network provider is available.

You can contact your state insurance department to find out if the nature of your complaint is eligible for review, or you can simply go ahead and file your grievance—if the state finds it ineligible for review, your appeal ends there. If it's found to merit a review, you'll need to submit the required paperwork.

What to Send

There's a reason why you need to keep copies of all your records and letters—because you'll need to submit all that paperwork from the internal review to the independent review:

- A letter from you explaining the situation. Be sure to address every point made by your insurance company and provide documentation to counter their arguments
- A letter of medical necessity (written by you or your child's doctor)
- A letter from your child's SLP explaining how therapy is helping your child
- Any supporting information, from books, articles, or reliable websites, on your child's particular diagnosis
- Copies of the rejected claims and the final determination not to provide coverage

Our pediatrician wrote a two-sentence letter of medical necessity, so I suspect it was my more detailed and impassioned letter that got us the coverage:

October 7, 2002

Appeals Section
Office of Financial and Insurance Services
P. O. Box XXXXX
Lansing, MI 48909

Re: Max

To Whom It May Concern:

This letter is to request an external review of [my insurance company] and their refusal to pay for speech therapy for my son, Max.

As you can see from the enclosed letter signed by Hearing Officer Lori B., the most recent rejection was the result of a managerial-level conference that included myself, my son's speech therapist Stephanie M., Ms. B., as well as a physician from the insurance company.

Ms. B. initially told me that a speech therapist would be participating in this conference—not a physician. I feel very strongly that a physician was not an appropriate professional to determine whether or not my child requires speech therapy, as most know nothing about my son's diagnosis of apraxia. My belief was proven correct when [my insurance company] offered this reason for rejection of payment: "our medical consultants reviewed the documentation . . . and confirmed that the apraxia is a developmental condition."

Apraxia is *not* a developmental condition. I am confident you will reach the same conclusion after you read the enclosed information.

When a condition is labeled "developmental," the implication is that the problem will eventually correct itself over time. A child with a developmental delay of speech is simply a child who is developing slower than what is considered normal. Also note that a child with a speech delay is more likely than not to be equally delayed in receptive and expressive speech; children with apraxia have no trouble with receptive language; it is only their expressive abilities that are severely limited.

We started speech therapy at the Kaufman Center in January 2002 when Max was two and a half years old. When most children this age have vocabularies of upwards of 100 words, Max had fewer than ten. He was incapable of imitating any words or sounds and would fly into a rage if asked to do so. He would smash his head into the floor from the frustration he felt knowing that he could not communicate his thoughts and that we had difficulty understanding him.

This speech problem affected far more than just Max's ability to communicate. It directly affected his behavior. He threw tantrums. He screamed. He smashed his head. He suffered from sensory issues, and simple tasks such as bathing and brushing teeth were ordeals for him. (Many kids with apraxia also suffer from sensory problems.) We couldn't take Max out shopping.

He was unable to sit in a restaurant for even half an hour. The behavioral problems were so unmanageable that I consulted a child psychologist. My own research led me to consider the possibility that Max was mildly autistic.

His problem all along was the apraxia.

Just one month of services at the Kaufman Center and Max became a different child. He could imitate words. He stopped throwing tantrums. He stopped smashing his head. He started talking in two- and three-word sentences. He can now string together up to fifteen words.

Here is what I need you to know: had Max never received speech therapy, he would still have that vocabulary of fewer than ten words. He never would have made any progress without the therapy because apraxia is not a simple delay.

Here is what else I need you to know: **if Max stops getting therapy, he will stop making progress**. As far as he has already come, he has a long way to go.

[My insurance company's] contract says it pays for speech services but not if the speech problem is a developmental condition. While apraxia is often called "developmental apraxia of speech," it is a neurological problem. I know it's confusing, but years ago when professionals were looking to give this condition a name, they realized it was much like the loss of speech that adults suffer from after a stroke. To differentiate apraxia in adults from apraxia in children, "developmental" was added to the diagnosis. It's not completely accurate.

The contract also says it will pay "for a condition that can be significantly improved in a reasonable and generally predictable period of time (usually about six months)." The language in this contract is vague and extremely subjective. Who's to say what is considered a "reasonable" amount of time? Max will probably need years of therapy. Given the nature of the problem, I consider that reasonable.

Given [my insurance company's] apparent lack of knowledge of apraxia I feel their rejection to cover therapy is inappropriate.

This request is in regards to rejected claims from Jan 2002 through March 2002. But I have speech therapy bills all the way through August 2002 that I have not yet submitted due to the past rejections. Therapy costs $60 per session and with an average of eight sessions a month, adds up to more than $400 a month.

This is not a minor situation by any means. I left my job in January 2002 in order to have the time to take Max to the five sessions a week of treatment he was requiring earlier this year. We have essentially slashed our income and greatly increased our expenses. My husband and I have turned our lives upside down to get Max the treatment he needs and deserves. Who would go through such a financial strain unless it was absolutely necessary?

I've enclosed copies of Max's evaluations and progress reports, as well as information from various sources on apraxia in general. I hope these help you in your review of my son's case. I appreciate your time and consideration and look forward to hearing from you soon.

Sincerely,

Debbie Feit

If the office finds the denied service is covered by your policy, your grievance gets the green light for a review. If it involves non-medical issues, it will most likely be reviewed by the state office. If it involves medical issues, it will get passed to an independent review organization. Insist that the right professional reviews your case. Most insurance companies will rely on doctors to review your case. But doctors are not the ones who provide speech therapy and they are not in a position to assess communication disorders and the necessary treatment. Request that an SLP review your case. If they won't honor your request, ask for a developmental pediatrician, who will be more knowledgeable about speech and language disorders than a general practice pediatrician.

DON'T GIVE UP THE FIGHT

I know that dealing with insurance companies and filing for appeals is a full-time job—one that you simply don't have time for. But if you're feeling that it's just not worth the hassle, consider this: A 2002 study of external review programs found that reviewers overturned denials an average of 45 percent across all states. (In some cases, the health plan reversed itself during the investigation.) So you're looking at some decent odds.

The entire insurance appeals process is set up to discourage you from fighting: The language in your plan may not be clear. It's almost impossible to work with the same agent from one phone call to the next, leaving you to start from the beginning each time. Your insurer may not inform you of your right to an appeal. There's tons of paperwork to manage and deadlines to meet. And with most states requiring that you exhaust the internal process before filing an external review, most parents are too exhausted to continue.

A 2002 study assessing external review programs in several states found that while appeals of medical necessity denials numbered in the thousands to tens of thousands, the number of consumers who applied for an external review only numbered in the dozens to hundreds.

Yes, the process is a pain. But by filing you'll not only help yourself, but other families as well. The state insurance offices keep data on the type of complaints that are filed. Having such information on the number of consumer complaints regarding speech therapy reimbursement will be valuable in national advocacy efforts working to improve coverage of speech therapy services.

12

The Tunnel Is Long, but I Promise There's a Light: Encouraging Advice, Words of Wisdom, and Happy Endings from Parents Just Like You

Max had been doing great in his three-year-old preschool class. Despite having an apraxia diagnosis, he was one of the most social and talkative kids in the class. But on a cold Thursday in December, during the preschool holiday concert, I would be faced with a reminder of Max's extensive problems—live and on stage.

The gym was filled with excited parents and apprehensive preschoolers. I made sure Max didn't see me when I took my seat because I feared he would come running to me, and I wanted to see him in the show.

What I saw made me want to cry. As soon as he took his seat on the bleachers, he started hitting and rubbing his eyes. I thought maybe he was having allergy problems, as it wasn't the first time I'd seen him rub his eyes. He just looked so uncomfortable.

When it was his class's turn to perform, he stood up, but he didn't sing. Was it stage fright? Or had he been unable to learn the words to the songs? Max just stood there looking alternately angry and lost. When I picked him up after class, I asked him about the show and told him I was there. He said, "No, I there." He either didn't understand what I was telling him or simply didn't want to acknowledge it.

I asked if it was scary, and he said yes. Then he volunteered that the reason he was hitting his face was so no one would take his picture. I hadn't even asked him about the hitting or the parents taking pictures. He brought it up on his own.

I know he doesn't always like people looking at him. But I don't know if that's a sensory thing or a control thing. Maybe it's just a Max thing.

Now I know what you're thinking—*this* is the light at the end of the tunnel? *This* is a success story?

Well, it's not. But before any of us can appreciate just how far our kids have come, we have to remind ourselves where they started. Up on those bleachers, surrounded by his fellow three- and four-year-olds singing "Rudolph the Red-Nosed Reindeer" to a crowded gym of grinning parents—we were only a few steps into that dark tunnel.

Exactly one year later . . . light.

It was once again time for the preschool holiday concert. Dave accompanied me this time, and from our seats we watched Max take his place in the front row. He and his classmates wore paper hats adorned with planet Earth. He waved to us and was all smiles. When it was another class's turn to sing "The Dreidel Song," Max happily—and loudly—joined in.

Despite sitting in the third row, Dave and I didn't have a great view of Max. So when it was time for his class to sing, Dave and I moved to stand along the side of the gym. Dave was videotaping so he didn't see the tears streaming down my face. Max was happily singing along, doing the accompanying hand gestures and occasionally arguing with the kid sitting behind him—he fit right in. I had never been so moved or felt so proud.

When we took our seats again I said to Dave, "Oh my God, I was crying back there." It was only then that I turned to look at him and I saw that Dave was crying, too! When we each saw the other crying, it only made us cry harder. We tried to divert the tears into laughter for fear that our fellow parents would think us nuts. Sure, it would have been natural for any parent to shed a few emotional tears of pride.

But Dave and I were sobbing with relief. Relief that, no matter how much more work lay ahead, Max would be OK in the end.

As of this writing, Max is seven years old and in the second grade. His apraxia was considered "resolved" by the time he started kindergarten, although he continued with speech therapy to help with resulting articulation issues. When he was five, he was diagnosed with ADHD, and speech therapy continued to play a vital role in his treatment. His therapists worked on his social language skills as well as addressing such areas as working memory, auditory processing, sequencing, and telling a narrative. Today he has an impressive vocabulary, an inquisitive mind, and a fabulously creative imagination. And he no longer requires speech therapy.

Ari, as of this writing, is five years old and in kindergarten. Her apraxia is, for the most part, "resolved," although she is experiencing some attentional and language-processing problems that we're still trying to sort through. She mixes up the words in her questions ("What that is?"), leaves out small words ("What Dad doing?"), and has trouble remembering things. Despite these difficulties, she started reading at age four and is quite skilled at writing and spelling. She emits a wonderful positive energy, loves learning, and has a willingness to try just about anything—other than new foods, that is.

I am not the only parent who has traveled down the road you are now starting. Nor am I the only one to eventually reach a wonderful destination.

"Austin is now six, and each year sees so much change and hope that it is hard to remember that when he was three and a half I didn't think he would ever be capable of going to kindergarten without an aide," says mom Renee. "I doubt I will ever be worry-free about his ability to take care of himself, but that is probably more of a parent issue as opposed to an apraxia one."

"I think only parents of children with speech and language issues can understand the high fives my husband and I gave each other when our son started saying 'no,' " says mom Frith. "Simple words that we take for granted in a toddler become huge milestones when those words took so long to arrive. Hopefully by kindergarten you won't be able to tell Decker was ever the silent little boy in playgroup from three years earlier."

"We are at the pool for swim lessons and the kids are taking turns being the caller for 'Red light, Green light,'" says mom Emily. "They call on Lillian—who mostly cannot talk in social situations—and I just about died. I was holding my breath and panicking as the other kids waited for her to start. She wasn't saying anything, so I call out to the instructor, 'She might want some help yelling,' and then all of a sudden Lillian calls out, 'Wed yite, gween yite!' I was beaming. I said, 'Can you believe it?' to the mom sitting next to me and she totally didn't get it."

That's not to say the journey is a smooth ride. There are often bumps. Sometimes it feels as if you are going in circles.

"Although Harley's struggles are at times oppressive and full of sadness, we thank God for sending him to us every day," says dad Jody. "He has taught us more about life and love in his thirteen years than we could possibly teach him in our combined lifetimes. Without him, we may have taken ourselves pretty darn seriously and ended up gliding through our days in a self-absorbed haze."

"I have always believed that it was good every now and then to take a week or so and just let myself feel bad. Feel sad. Feel mad," says mom Sharon. "I find there is a synchronicity to this. Landmark occasions tended to set it off—birthdays, new school years. But inevitably, and always, I knew I had to lift myself up, brush myself off, breathe, and go on. I not only had to secure the best services that actually met Luke's needs, but I needed to be his voice in the world until he could have his own voice."

"The never-ending process of evaluations and therapy is draining," says mom Susan. "It seems every time I get excited about my daughter's progress, BAM! It's time for yet another evaluation and yet another wave of anxiety and sadness about how others perceive Allison; where they think she is in her speech and related development, and how far they think she has to go."

Parent to Parent

I knew everything would be OK when . . .

- "He went from that first 'mama' to twenty or so words in a matter of weeks."
- "She went from just a few sounds and about 200 signs to talking in sentences when prompted—and sometimes when not. This was after being told by her neurologist that there was a 50 percent chance she wouldn't talk."
- "Everyone could understand him. I knew the rest of the way would be downhill."
- "He woke in the middle of the night, pointed to his ear and said, 'I have owie in my ear. My ear hurts. Make boo boo in ear go away, Mommy.' This was the first time Decker had ever been able to communicate to us what exactly felt wrong when he was sick. My heart sank knowing he was in pain, but it was also flying because he was able to do more than whimper and cry in discomfort."
- "Without realizing it, I found I was able to understand Jordan much more and I wasn't translating for others. This really snuck up on me."
- "I realized that Maya is aware that she has a different learning style but she still feels great about herself and is motivated to learn and work."
- "After two years of unproductive therapy, his therapist at the Mayo Clinic had him saying 'me' after about three minutes of working with him."
- "She was finally able to correctly repeat 'bye-bye' instead of saying 'die-die.' Now people knew she was being social and not wishing death upon them."
- "I heard her mimic her first multisyllabic word—lollipop."
- "Two mothers from school called to say their sons were begging for a playdate with Sam. I nearly cried. That was better proof of his progress than anything else."

(continued on next page)

> • "After watching a *Signing Time* video he was able to repeat every sign he saw two hours later. It was the first time I could say for certain that he had the words in his head. We just had to find a way to get them out."

"We are so lucky to have James in our lives," says mom Charlotte. "He's taught us compassion, patience, empathy, and love of children who are special. Our oldest son grows and develops normally and we've never had real challenges with him. With James, we do. And our life is richer for it."

FINAL WORDS OF WISDOM

You may meet one, or several, professionals on this journey to help your child communicate. Some will be helpful; others will not. But one thing is true—the *parents* you meet along the way will always have wisdom to share. Here's what the ones interviewed for this book had to offer in the way of parting advice:

- "Do not settle for a 'global delay' or 'speech delay' diagnosis. Fight for finding out exactly what the problem is. Get the specific help your child needs and do not be afraid to buck the system to get it! Do this while your child is still young. Don't wait around."
- "Realize that the start of the process is just that—a start. There's a lot more to come. Focus on the fact that you've taken the first step, which is the best thing you can do for your child."
- "You are blessed. It won't always feel like a blessing when you're on the phone fighting with the insurance company or in the hospital for another test. I personally feel honored to raise one of these precious souls."
- "Get help from those who listen to you and your concerns. Yes, the speech therapy is for your child. But you also need support

and if you don't feel taken care of, go elsewhere. You need to feel good about the services provided."

- "Your child is your child . . . she isn't her disability."
- "Look at the process one step at a time. It is entirely doable."
- "Make sure all your waking moments are not spent overanalyzing what your child is doing or what the tests said. I used to keep a journal of things I saw my son do and where he was improving. It was getting out of hand. Most parents jot down major milestones. I was writing a novel. You have to let your child be."
- "Take every day, every therapy session, and realize you are moving forward. Accept that it may be slow, and don't give it a timeline for resolution. As long as your child is making strides you are moving in the right direction."

No matter where you and your child may be on your journey, know that you will see progress. It may not be quick. It may not be easy. And for every two steps forward, your child may take one step back. But with the right treatment from a skilled professional—and support from you and your family—your child's speech and language skills can improve.

Every child comes with his or her own unique set of challenges. Some may need braces or a math tutor. Others may need to be more responsible with their toys or less sensitive about getting their feelings hurt. Our kids need help with their communication. And it is our job to provide them with the support they need. It is also our job—and this part can be far more difficult—to accept our children's differences.

Yes, it's important to understand their speech or language problem and to get them the appropriate treatment. But once therapy is under way, and we have been equipped with the necessary tools to help our child at home, we must try to just let things be. Not every interaction with our child has to be a therapeutic opportunity. Kids need the time and space to simply be—and it's our job to give them that, too.

This journey through the tunnel is not always an express trip. Some days you'll take pleasure in the smooth ride. Others, you may find yourself lost; you may feel impatient and frustrated. I hope this book will prove to be your trusty guide and provide you with the information and support you need. And remember—as long as you keep moving, you will reach the light at the end.

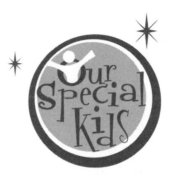

Because parents of special needs kids have needs, too.
www.ourspecialkids.com

Please let us know how this book has helped you. Contact the authors at debbie@ourspecialkids.com.

For more information on raising a child with special needs, please visit ourspecialkids.com, where you'll find a sense of community, a wealth of resources, and the opportunity to share your child's latest success.

Bibliography

Adams, Catherine, Julian Lloyd, Catherine Aldred, and Janet Baxendale. "Exploring the Effects of Communication Intervention for Developmental Pragmatic Language Impairments." *International Journal of Language and Communication Disorders*, 41 (1) 41–65, January/February 2006.

Agin, Marilyn C. "Apraxia, What's That?" Presented at the First Conference for Verbal Apraxia, Morristown, NJ, July 23–24, 2001.

Agin, Marilyn C., Lisa F. Geng, and Malcolm J. Nicholl, *The Late Talker: What to Do If Your Child Isn't Talking Yet.* New York: St. Martin's Press, 2003.

Agin, Marilyn C., Robert Katz, and Lori L. Roth. "Verbal Apraxia/Dyspraxia and the Therapeutic Role of Essential Fatty Acids." Presented at the First Conference for Verbal Apraxia, Morristown, NJ, July 23–24, 2001.

Aguilar, B., L. A. Sroufe, B. Egeland, and E. Carlson, "Distinguishing the Early-Onset/Persistent and Adolescence-Onset Antisocial Behavior Types: From Birth to 16 Years." *Development and Psychopathology*, vol. 12, 109–132, 2000.

Alvord, Becky. Interview. January 23, 2007.

American Academy of Child and Adolescent Psychiatry. "The Child and Adolescent Psychiatrist." aacap.org.

———. "Comprehensive Psychiatric Evaluation." aacap.org.

American Academy of Otolaryngology—Head and Neck Surgery. "What Is an Otolaryngologist?" entnet.org

American Academy of Pediatrics. "Complementary and Alternative Medicine." aap.org.

———. "Television and the Family." aap.org.

American Association on Mental Retardation. "Fact Sheet: Frequently Asked Questions About Mental Retardation." aamr.org.

American Hippotherapy Association. "Introduction to Hippotherapy." americanhippotherapyassociation.org.

American Occupational Therapy Association. "Occupational Therapy for Children." aota.org.

———. "What Is Occupational Therapy?" aota.org.

American Speech–Language–Hearing Association. "Acquiring English as a Second Language." Rockville, MD: ASHA, 2005.

———. "Activities to Encourage Speech and Language Development." Rockville, MD: ASHA, 2005.

———. "Auditory Integration Training." Position Statement, 2004.

————. "Auditory Processing Disorder." Rockville, MD: ASHA, 2005.

————. "Causes of Hearing Loss in Children." Rockville, MD: ASHA, 2005.

————. "(Central) Auditory Processing Disorders. Technical Report." Rockville, MD: ASHA, 2005.

————. "Childhood Apraxia of Speech." Rockville, MD: ASHA, 2005.

————. "Children and Bilingualism." Rockville, MD: ASHA, 2005.

————. "Dysarthria." Rockville, MD: ASHA, 2005.

————. "Effects of Hearing Loss on Development." Rockville, MD: ASHA, 2005.

————. "How Does Your Child Hear and Talk?" Rockville, MD: ASHA, 2005.

————. "Introduction to Augmentative and Alternative Communication." Rockville, MD: ASHA, 2005.

————. "Late Blooming or Language Problem?" Rockville, MD: ASHA, 2005.

————. "Making Sense of Your Health Insurance Plan." Rockville, MD: ASHA, 2005.

————. "Obtaining Reimbursement for Stuttering Treatment." Rockville, MD: ASHA, 2005.

————. "Pragmatic Language Tips." Rockville, MD: ASHA, 2005.

————. "Pragmatics, Socially Speaking." Rockville, MD: ASHA, 2005.

————. "Private Health Plans." Rockville, MD: ASHA, 2005.

————."Speech Language Pathology: Nature of the Work." Rockville, MD: ASHA, 2005.

————. "Type, Degree and Configuration of Hearing Loss." Rockville, MD: ASHA, 2005.

————. "What Is Stuttering?" Rockville, MD: ASHA, 2005.

ASHA *Leader Online.* "Getting Health Plans to Pay for Pediatric Verbal Apraxia." asha.org.

Annandale Fluency Clinic. "Information Sheet for Parents of Young School-Aged Children Who Stutter." afccafet.com.

Apel, Kenn, and Julie J. Masterson. *Beyond Baby Talk: From Sounds to Sentences— A Parent's Complete Guide to Language Development.* Roseville, CA: Prima, 2001.

Arc of Minnesota. "Waivered Services." thearcofminnesota.org.

Astington, J. W., and J. M. Jenkins. "A Longitudinal Study of the Relation Between Language and Theory-of-Mind Development." *Developmental Psychology,* 35, 1311–1320, 1999.

"Autism and the Gluten-Free/Casein-Free Diet: A Guide for Parents, Dieticians and Other Health Professionals." glutenfree.com.

Autism Society of America. "Defining Autism." autism-society.org.

————. "Dietary Interventions." autism-society.org.

Autistic Continuum Connections, Education, and Support Site. "Nonverbal Learning Disability." access.autistics.org.

Beitchman, J. H., R. Nair, M. Clegg, et al. "Prevalence of Psychiatric Disorders in Children with Speech and Language Disorders." *Journal of the American Academy of Child and Adolescent Psychiatry,* 25, 528–535, 1986.

Beitchman, J. H., B. Wilson, E. B. Brownlie, et al. "Long-Term Consistency in Speech/Language Profiles II. Behavioral, Emotional and Social Outcomes." *Journal of the American Academy of Child and Adolescent Psychiatry*, 36 (6), 815–825, 1996.

Bell, Kay. "IRS Approved Limited Carryover of FSA Balance." bankrate.com.

Berk, L. E. "Children's Private Speech." *Private Speech: From Social Interaction to Self-Regulation*. L. E. Berk and R. M. Diaz (Eds.) Hillside, NJ: Erlbaum, 1992.

Blatchford, P. "Academic Self-Assessment at 7 and 11 Years: Its Accuracy and Association with Ethnic Group and Sex." *British Journal of Educational Psychology*, 62, 35–44, 1992.

Bloch, Sally. Interview. November 6, 2006.

Borzo, Greg. "Horse Power: Hippotherapy Has Begun to Attract Attention from the Medical Community. One Physician Even Owns His Own Program." *American Medical News*, vol. 45, no. 23, 24 (3), June 17, 2002.

Bothe, Anne Cordes. "Parents as Partners in Young Children's Stuttering Treatment." Minnesota State University. mnsu.edu.

Bowen, Caroline. "Tongue-Tie." speech-language-therapy.com.

———. "Developmental Apraxia of Speech: Information for Families." speech-language-therapy.com.

———. "Frequently Asked Questions About Speech-Language Pathology." speech-language-therapy.com.

———. "Modeling and Recasting—Facilitating Language Learning." speech-language-therapy.com.

———. "Oral Motor Exercises: Why Not?" speech-language-therapy.com.

———. "Semantic and Pragmatic Difficulties." speech-language-therapy.com.

———. "Traditional Articulation Therapy." speech-language-therapy.com.

———. "Voice Therapy for Children." speech-language-therapy.com.

———. "What Is the Evidence for Oral Motor Therapy?" *Acquiring Knowledge in Speech, Language and Hearing*, vol. 7, no. 3, 2005.

———. *Developmental Phonological Disorders: A Practical Guide for Families and Teachers*. Melbourne, Australia: The Australia Council for Educational Research Ltd, 1998.

Bowen, Caroline, and Linda Cupples. "PACT: Parents and Children Together in Phonological Therapy." *Advances in Speech Language Pathology*, vol. 8, no. 3, 282–292, 2006.

Boys Town National Research Hospital. "My Baby's Hearing." babyhearing.org.

Brain Tumor Foundation for Children. "The Difference Between Speech and Language," btfcgainc.org.

Bristol, M. M. "Mothers of Children with Autism or Communication Disorders: Successful Adaptation and the Double ABCX Model." *Journal of Autism and Developmental Disabilities*, vol. 17, no. 4, December 1987.

Bristol, M., J. Gallagher, and E. Schopler. "Mothers and Fathers of Young Developmentally Disabled and Nondisabled Boys: Adaptation and Spousal Support." *Developmental Psychology*, 24, 441–451, 1988.

Brown, Frank R., III, Elizabeth H. Aylward, and Barbara K. Keogh. "The Relationship Between Language and Learning Difficulties." ldonline.org.

———. *Diagnosis and Management of Learning Disabilities: An Interdisciplinary/Lifespan Approach*, Third Edition. Belmont, CA: Thomson Wadsworth, 1996.

Brownlie, E. B. "Early Language Impairment and Young Adult Delinquent and Aggressive Behavior." *Journal of Abnormal Psychology*, August 2004.

Bruder, Mary Beth. "The Individual Family Service Plan." Education Resources Information Center. ericdigests.org.

Burns, R. *Self-Concept Development and Education*. London, England: Holt, Rinehart and Winston, 1982.

Burns, Tim. "How Parents Can Help Their Child with Apraxia at Home." apraxia-kids.org.

C. S. Mott Children's Hospital, University of Michigan Health System. "Speech Problems: Normal vs. Stuttering." med.umich.edu.

Chapman, J. W. "Learning Disabled Children's Self Concept." *Review of Educational Research*, 58, 347–371, 1988.

Childhood Apraxia of Speech Association of North America. "What Is Childhood Apraxia of Speech?" apraxia-kids.org.

———. "How State Insurance Commissions Can Help with Insurance Funding." apraxia-kids.org.

———. "Insurance Tips for Families." apraxia-kids.org.

Children and Adults with Attention Deficit/Hyperactivity Disorder (CHADD). "The Disorder Named AD/HD: CHADD Fact Sheet #1." chadd.org.

———. "Assessing Complementary and/or Controversial Interventions: CHADD Fact Sheet #6." chadd.org.

Children's Hospital Boston. "Neuro Examination." childrenshospital.org.

Cici, Regina. *What's Wrong with Me? Learning Disabilities at Home and School.* Baltimore, MD: York Press, 1995.

Cincinnati Children's Hospital. "Articulation." cincinnatichildrens.org.

———. "Language Disorder." cincinnatichildrens.org.

———. "Stuttering." cincinnatichildrens.org.

———. "Voice." cincinnatichildrens.org.

City University of New York, The Graduate Center. "Specific Language Impairment."

Cleveland, Sandra. "Central Auditory Processing Disorder: When Is Evaluation Referral Indicated?" ldonline.org.

Clopton, James R., and Jennifer L. Boothe. "How Parenting Children with Special Needs Influences the Marital Relationship." *S.I. Focus*, Autumn 2005.

Close, Robin. "Television and Language Development in the Early Years: A Review of the Literature." The National Literacy Trust. literacytrust.org.uk.

Cohen, N. J., R. Menna, D. D. Vallance, et al. "Language, Social Cognitive Processing, and Behavioral Characteristics of Psychiatrically Disturbed Children with Previously Identified and Unsuspected Language Impairments." *Journal of Child Psychology and Psychiatry*, 39, 853–864, 1998.

Committee on Children with Disabilities of the American Academy of Pediatrics. "Developmental Surveillance and Screening of Infants and Young Children." *Pediatrics*, vol. 108, no. 1, 192–195, July 2001.

Congress of Neurological Surgeons. "Cranial Nerves." neurosurgeon.org.

Consumers Union. "A Consumer Guide to Handling Disputes with Your Employer or Private Health Plan." 2005. consumersunion.org.

Cook, Gretchen. "Siblings of Disabled Have Their Own Troubles." *New York Times*, April 4, 2006.

Councill, Ellen. "Speech and Language Terms or 'Speech Therapy 101'." apraxia-kids.org.

Daily Routines for Parents and Professionals: Preschool. East Moline, IL: LinguiSystems, Inc., 1999.

Desjarlais, Roy. Interview. August 4, 2006.

Dismuke-Blakely, Ruth. Interview. July 28, 2006.

———. "Hippotherapy As a Treatment Strategy in Speech and Language Remediation." American Hippotherapy Association. Level 1 Treatment Principles Workshop Manual, First Edition. AHA, Inc. 2006.

Early On Michigan. Michigan Department of Education. "Michigan's Family Guidebook to Early Intervention Services," 1993.

Edelen-Smith, P. J. "How Now Brown Cow: Phoneme Awareness Activities for Collaborative Classrooms." *Intervention in School and Clinic*, vol. 33, no. 2, 103–111, 1997.

Edelson, Meredyth Goldberg. "Social Stories." Center for the Study of Autism. autism.org.

Edelson, Stephen M. "Leaky Gut and the Gluten-/Casein-Free Diet." Center for the Study of Autism. autism.org.

Ellis, Edwin S. "How Now Brown Cow: Phoneme Awareness Activities." ldonline.org.

"Essential Fatty Acids." *Encyclopedia of Alternative Medicine*. Thomson Gale, 2006. health.enotes.com.

"Expressive Language Disorder." *Encyclopedia of Mental Disorders*. minddisorders.com.

Family Voices. "Beginning the Conversation: A Report of Family Voices' Interview with Seventeen Managed Care Organizations." November 2001. familyvoices.org.

Feit, Debbie. "Learning to Talk." *Parents*, February, 2005.

Feldman, Heidi M., and Cheryl Messick. "Assessment of Language and Speech." *Developmental and Behavioral Pediatrics*. M. L. Wolraich, P. H. Dworkin, D. D. Drotar, and E. Perrin (Eds.). Philadelphia: Elsevier, 2007.

Feldscher, Karen. " 'Miracle' Treatment for Autism May Be Dangerous." *The Northeastern Voice*, May 16, 1996.

Freinkel, Susan. "Uncomfortable in Their Own Skin." alternativemedicine.com.

Frick, Sheila and Hacker, Colleen. "Auditory Interventions: What's Right for My Child?" NeuroTherapeutics, Inc. nt4kids.com.

Gillam, Ronald B., Diane Frome Loeb, and Sandy Friel-Patti. "Looking Back: A Summary of Five Exploratory Studies of Fast ForWord." *American Journal of Speech-Language Pathology*, vol. 10, 269–273, August 2001.

Glascoe, Frances P., and Henry L. Shapiro, "Introduction to Developmental and Behavioral Screening." Developmental Behavioral Pediatrics Online. dbpeds.org.

Glennen, Sharon. "Language Development and Delay in Internationally Adopted Infants and Toddlers: A Review." *American Journal of Speech-Language Pathology*, vol. 11, 333–339, November 2002.

Golden, Ellen. "Voice Disorders in Children." The Center for Speech, Language and Occupational Therapy. cslot.com.

Goldstein, Brian. Interview. June 25, 2006.

Golinkoff, Roberta Michnick, and Kathy Hirsh-Pasek. *How Babies Talk: The Magic and Mystery of Language in the First Three Years of Life*. New York: Plume, 2000.

Green, Carolyn, Craig W. Martin, Ken Bassett, and Arminée Kazanjian. "A Systematic Review and Critical Appraisal of the Scientific Evidence on Craniosacral Therapy." Joint Health Technology Assessment Series. British Columbia Office of Health Technology Assessment. May 1999.

Greenspan, Stanley. Interview. August 5, 2006.

Gretz, Sharon. "How to Think About a Speech/Language Evaluation." Apraxia-Kids. apraxia-kids.org.

———. "Because It's Your Child! Evaluating Information on the Internet." Apraxia-Kids. apraxia-kids.org.

———. Interview. March 24, 2003.

———. "Literacy and Children with Apraxia of Speech." Apraxia-Kids. apraxia-kids.org.

Halfon, Neal, Miles Hochstein, Harvinder Sareen, et al. "Barriers to the Provision of Developmental Assessments During Pediatric Health Supervision." Presented at the Pediatric Academic Societies annual meeting, May 2001.

Hamaguchi, Patricia McAleer. *Childhood Speech, Language and Listening Problems: What Every Parent Should Know*. New York: John Wiley & Sons, 2001.

Hamilton, L., D. Keating, S. McMahon, and M. Syrmis. "Pediatricians: Referral Rates and Speech Pathology Waiting Lists." *Journal of Pediatrics and Child Health*, vol. 5, 451–455, 1998.

Hammer, David. "Brief Ideas for Speech Therapy for Children with Apraxia of Speech." apraxia-kids.org.

Harrington, Jonathan, and Mannell, Robert. "Distinctive Features." MacQuarie University, Sydney, Australia. ling.mq.edu.au.

Hill, Jennifer. Interview. April 1, 2006.

———. Interview. June 20, 2006.

———. Interview. August 15, 2006.

Hodge, Megan. "What is Neuroplasticity and Why Do Parents and SLPs Need to Know?" Apraxia-Kids. apraxia-kids.org

Hume-O'Haire, Elizabeth, and Stephen Winters. "Distinctive Feature Theory." *The Encyclopedia of Cognitive Science.* London, England: MacMillian, 2002.

"Hypotonia." *Encyclopedia of Children's Health.* healthofchildren.com.

"IEP Goals and Objectives Bank." Bend Lapine Schools. Bend, OR, 2006.

Innis, Sheila M. "Perinatal Biochemistry and Physiology of Long-Chain Polyunsaturated Fatty Acids." *Journal of Pediatrics,* 143, S1–8, October 2003.

Innis, Sheila M., Judith Gilley, and Janet Werker. "Are Human Milk Long-Chain Polyunsaturated Fatty Acids Related to Visual and Neural Development in Breast-Fed Term Infants?" *Journal of Pediatrics,* vol. 139, no. 4, October 2001.

Innovative Therapies. "Therapeutic Listening." innovative-therapies.com.

Interactive Metronome. "Neurological and Motor Rehabilitation Overview." interactivemetronome.com.

International Alliance of Health Care Educators. "Craniosacral Therapy/ SomatoEmotional Release." iahe.com.

Jakielski, Kathy, Thomas P. Marquardt, and Barbara L. Davis. "Developmental Apraxia of Speech: Information for Parents." Apraxia-Kids. apraxia-kids.org.

Kaiser Family Foundation. "Assessing State External Review Programs and the Effects of Pending Federal Patients' Rights Legislation." March 2002. kff.org.

Kaufman Children's Center for Speech, Language, Sensory-Motor, and Social Connections. "Signs and Symptoms: Expressive Language Disorders/ Receptive Language Disorders." kidspeech.com.

———. "Helping the Child with Apraxia of Speech." kidspeech.com.

———. "Sensory Integration." kidspeech.com.

———. "Signs and Symptoms: Autism." kidspeech.com.

———. "Signs and Symptoms: Apraxia." kidspeech.com.

———. "Signs and Symptoms: Social Pragmatic Language Disorder." kidspeech.com.

———. "What Is Craniosacral Therapy?" kidspeech.com.

Kaufman, Nancy. Interview. November 10, 2005.

———. Interview. June 25, 2006.

Kentucky Children's Hospital. "Vocal Cord Disorders." ukhealthcare.uky.edu.

KidSource Online. "What is Early Intervention?" kidsource.com.

Knivsberg, A. M., K. L. Reichelt, and M. Nodland. "Reports on Dietary Intervention in Autistic Disorders." *Nutritional Neuroscience,* 4(1): 25–37, 2001.

Koomar, Jane, Jeanetta D. Burpee, Valerie DeJean, et al. "Theoretical and Clinical Perspectives on the Interactive Metronome: A View From Occupational Therapy Practice." *American Journal of Occupational Therapy,* vol. 55, no. 2, March/April 2001.

Kranowitz, Carol Stock. *The Out-of-Sync Child: Recognizing and Coping with Sensory Integration Dysfunction.* New York: Perigee, 1998.

Kuhlthau, Karen, Kristen Smith Hill, Recai Yucel, and James M. Perrin. "Financial Burden for Families of Children with Special Health Care Needs." *Maternal and Child Health Journal,* vol. 9, no. 2, June 2005.

Kutscher, Martin L. *ADHD Book: Living Right Now!* White Plains, NY: Neurology Press, 2004.

Language Express Preschool Speech Language Service System (Ontario). "Problem Voice?" language-express.ca.

Lawrence, Michael, and David M. Barclay III. "Stuttering: A Brief Review." *American Family Physician*, May 1, 1998.

Lindsay, Geoff, and Julie Dockrell. "The Behavior and Self-Esteem of Children with Specific Speech and Language Difficulties." *British Journal of Educational Psychology*, 70, 583–601, 2000.

Liss, Barry D. Interview. October 6, 2006.

Little Works in Progress Pediatric Therapy. "Speech Therapy and Occupational Therapy." littleworksinprogress.com.

Lobato, Debra, and Barbara Kao. "Family-Based Group Intervention for Young Siblings of Children with Chronic Illness and Developmental Disability." *Journal of Pediatric Psychology*, 30, 678–682, December 2005.

Lof, Gregory L. "What Does the Research Say Regarding Oral Motor Exercises and the Treatment of Speech Sound Disorders?" apraxia-kids.org.

———."Logic, Theory and Evidence Against the Use of Non-Speech Oral Motor Exercises to Change Speech Sound Productions." Presented at the American Speech-Language-Hearing Association Convention, Miami Beach, FL, 2006.

Lucker-Lazerson, Nancy. "Apraxia? Dyspraxia? Articulation? Phonology? What Does It All Mean?" Apraxia-Kids. apraxia-kids.org.

Macauley, Beth L. Letter to the editor. *The ASHA Leader*, December 16, 2003.

Maine Consumer Guide to Health Insurers, 2005. maine.gov.

March of Dimes. "Down Syndrome." marchofdimes.com.

Marshak, Laura E., and Fran Pollock-Prezant. *Married with Special-Needs Children: A Couples' Guide to Keeping Connected.* Bethesda, MD: Woodbine House, 2006.

Martin, Allison. "Your Adopted Child's Speech and Language Development." *Adoptive Families*, November/December 2003.

Martin, Katherine L. *Does My Child Have a Speech Problem?* Chicago: Chicago Review Press, 1997.

Maryland Insurance Administration's 2003 Report on the Health Care Appeals and Grievance Law, August 2004.

McCaffrey, Patrick. "Dysarthria: Characteristics, Prognosis, Remediation." California State University. csuchico.edu.

———. "Neuropathologies of Swallowing and Speech." California State University. csuchico.edu.

McCarty, Janet P. Interview. October 4, 2006.

McCarty, Janet P., Maureen E. Thompson, and Steven C. White. *Appealing Health Plan Denials.* Rockville, Maryland: American Speech-Language-Hearing Association, 2002.

"Medical Specialists: Developmental Pediatrician." wrongdiagnosis.com.

Midland County Educational Service Agency. "Therapeutic Listening." mcesa.k12.mi.us.

Moore, Kent J. "Navigating the Patient Appeals Process." *Family Practice Management*, vol. 7, no. 9, October 2000.

Morales, Sarah. "Expressive Language Disorder." Children's Speech Care Center. childspeech.net.

Nancarrow, Diane. Interview. March 8, 2006.

Nathan, Liz, Joy Stackhouse, and Nata Goulandris. "The Development of Early Literacy Skills Among Children with Speech Difficulties." *Journal of Speech, Language and Hearing Research*, vol. 47, 377–391, April 2004.

National Association for the Self-Employed. "Health Insurance Help." health.nase.org.

National Center for Complementary and Alternative Medicine, National Institute of Health. "What is Complementary and Alternative Medicine?" nccam.nih.gov.

———. "10 Things to Know About Evaluating Medical Resources on the Web." nccam.nih.gov.

National Center of Medical Home Initiatives for Children with Special Needs. "Newborn and Infant Hearing Screening Activities." medicalhomeinfo.org.

———. "What is a Medical Home?" medicalhomeinfo.org.

National Center on Low-Incidence Disabilities. "Pop-up IEP for Parents/ Advocates." nclid.unco.edu.

National Dissemination Center for Children with Disabilities. "Questions Often Asked by Parents About Special Education Services." nichcy.org.

———. "Developing Your Child's IEP." nichcy.org.

———. "Mental Retardation." Disability Fact Sheet.

———. "Your Child's Education." nichcy.org.

National Down Syndrome Congress. "Facts About Down Syndrome." ndsccenter.org.

National Information Center for Children and Youth with Disabilities. "Children with Disabilities: Understanding Sibling Issues." *NICHCY News Digest*, no. 11, 1988.

National Institute on Deafness and Other Communication Disorders. "Speech and Language: Developmental Milestones." nidcd.nih.gov.

———. "Apraxia of Speech." nidcd.nih.gov.

———. "Auditory Processing Disorder in Children." nidcd.nih.gov.

———. "Autism and Communication." nidcd.nih.gov.

———. "Disorders of Vocal Abuse." nidcd.nih.gov.

———. "Stuttering." nidcd.nih.gov.

———. "What Is Voice? What Is Speech? What Is Language?" nidcd.nih.gov.

National Institute of Neurological Disorders and Stroke. "Infantile Hypotonia Information Page." ninds.nih.gov.

National Library of Medicine. "Phonological Disorder." nlm.nih.gov.

National Stuttering Association. "Insurance Advocacy and Stuttering." nsastutter.org.

———. "Overview of Speech Therapy for Teenagers Who Stutter." nsastutter.org.

New Jersey Speech-Hearing-Language Association. "What Is Voice?" njsha.org.

New York State Department of Health, Early Intervention Program. *Clinical Practice Guideline: Report of the Recommendations.* Communication Disorders, Assessment and Intervention for Young Children (Age 0–3 Years). Albany, NY: New York State Department of Health, 1999.

———. *Clinical Practice Guideline: The Guideline Technical Report.* Communications Disorders, Assessment and Intervention for Young Children (Age 0–3 Years). Albany, NY: New York State Department of Health, 1999.

New York University Child Study Center. "Central Auditory Processing Disorder." aboutourkids.org.

Nolan, Lea. "What I Learned Fighting My Insurance Company . . . or Keys to Successfully Aquiring Speech Therapy Services Through a Managed Care Organization." apraxia-kids.org.

Nonverbal Learning Disorders Association. "Nonverbal Learning Disabilities." nlda.org.

Novak, Maria. "How to Find a Speech Language Pathologist." apraxia-kids.org.

Ohio Speech-Language-Hearing Association. "Insurance Tips." ohioslha.org.

Olswang, Lesley B., Barbara Rodriguez, and Geralyn Timler. "Recommending Intervention for Toddlers with Specific Language Learning Difficulties: We May Not Have All the Answers, but We Know a Lot." *American Journal of Speech-Language Pathology*, 7:23–32, February 1998.

"Overview of Special Education Law." nolo.com.

Owens, Robert E., Dale Evan Metz, and Adelaide Haas. *Introduction to Communication Disorders: A Life Span Perspective*, Second Edition. Boston: Allyn and Bacon, 2003.

Pancsofar, Nadya, and Lynne Vernon-Feagans. "Mother and Father Language Input to Young Children: Contributions to Later Language Development." *Journal of Applied Developmental Psychology*, November/December 2006.

Parent Advocacy Coalition for Educational Rights. "What Is the Difference Between an IFSP and an IEP?" pacer.org.

Paton, Judith W. "Central Auditory Processing Disorders." Learning Disabilities Online. ldonline.org.

Patterson, G. R. *Coercive Family Interactions.* Eugene, OR: Castalia Press, 1982.

"Pediatric Voice Disorders." voiceproblem.org.

Pennsylvania Speech-Language-Hearing Association. "Insurance Appeal on Behalf of a Child with Apraxia." *Keystater*, September 1992.

Perry, Patrick. "Battling the Blues: Ongoing Research Shows that Omega-3 Fatty Acids Help Treat Depression: An Interview with Andrew Stoll, MD. *Saturday Evening Post*, May/June 2005.

Pine, D. S., G. E. Bruder, G. A. Wasserman, et al. "Verbal Dichotic Listening in Boys at Risk for Behavior Disorders." *Journal of the American Academy of Child and Adolescent Psychiatry*, vol. 36, 1465–1473, 1997.

Ping, Liew. "Choosing Specialist Services for Your Child." web.singnet.com. sg/~liewping/index.html.

Pollock-Prezant, Fran. Interview. October 19, 2006.

Powell, T. H., and P. A. Ogle, *Brothers and Sisters: A Special Part of Exceptional Families*. Baltimore: Paul H. Brookes, 1985.

Prader-Willi Syndrome Association. "Speech and Language and Prader-Willi Syndrome." pwsausa.org.

Princeton Speech-Language and Learning Center. "Articulation Disorders." psllcnj.com.

Quest Diagnostics. "Speech and Language Development." questdiagnostics.com.

Ramsey, Mariann. Interview. June 19, 2006.

Rankovic, Christine M., William M. Rabinowitz, and Gregory L. Lof. "Maximum Output Intensity of the Audiokinetron." *American Journal of Speech-Language Pathology*, vol. 5, 68–72, May 1996.

"Receptive Language Disorder." Department of Human Services, Victoria, Australia. betterhealthchannel.vic.gov.au.

Redmond, S. M., and M. L. Rice. "The Socioemotional Behaviors of Children with Specific Language Impairment: Social Adaptation or Social Deviance?" *Journal of Speech, Language and Hearing Research*, 41, 688–700, 1998.

Remenar, Kristen. "Children's Book Reviews." ourspecialkids.com

Rentschler, Gary J. "Stuttering Therapy." home.duq.edu/~rentschler.

Rhode Island Hospital. "Brothers and Sisters of Children with Disabilities: Guidelines for Parents." lifespan.org.

———. "Helping Siblings of Children with Disabilities." lifespan.org.

Richardson, Alexandra J. "Dyslexia, Dyspraxia and ADHD—Can Nutrition Help?" apraxia-kids.org.

Romaniec, Mary. "Closing the Deal: A Street-Smart Approach to Negotiating Your Child's IEP." *Autism Asperger's Digest*, March/April 2005.

Rosenfield, David B. "Do Stutterers Have Different Brains?" *Neurology*, 57, 171–172, 2001.

Rosin, Peggy. Interview. July 5, 2006.

Rosin, Peggy, and Giuliana Miolo. "Improving Communication Skills of Children with Down Syndrome." Two-day workshop. Madison, WI. October 13–14, 2005.

Roth, Froma P., and Colleen K. Worthington. *Treatment Resource Manual for Speech-Language Pathology*, Third Edition. Thomson Delmar Learning, 2005.

Rudolph, Michael, Frank Rosanowski, Ulrich Eysholdt, and Peter Kummer. "Anxiety and Depression in Mothers of Speech Impaired Children." *International Journal of Pediatric Otorhinolaryngology*, 67, 1337–1341, 2003.

———. "Quality of Life in Mothers of Speech Impaired Children." *Logopedics Phoniatrics Vocology*, 30, 3–8, 2005.

Rvachew, Susan, and Meghann Grawburg. "Correlates of Phonological Awareness in Preschoolers with Speech Sound Disorders." *Journal of Speech, Language and Hearing Research*, vol. 49, 74–87, February 2006.

Sander, E. K. "When Are Speech Sounds Learned?" *Journal of Speech and Hearing Disorders*, 37: 55–63, 1972.

Sanders, Heather, Melinda F. Davis, Burris Duncan, et al. "Use of Complementary and Alternative Therapies Among Children with Special Health Care Needs in Southern Arizona." *Pediatrics*, vol. III, no. 3, 584–587, March 2003.

Schwartz, Sue. *The New Language of Toys: Teaching Communication Skills to Children with Special Needs*, Third Edition. Bethesda, MD: Woodbine House, 2004.

Schwartz, Susan J. "Central Auditory Processing Disorder." Child Study Center, New York University School of Medicine. aboutourkids.org.

Scott, David T., Jeri S. Janowsky, Robin E. Carroll, et al. "Formula Supplementation with Long-Chain Polyunsaturated Fatty Acids: Are There Developmental Benefits?" *Pediatrics*, vol.102, no. 5, E59, November 1998.

Seltzer, M., J. Greenberg, F. Floyd, et al. "Life Course Impacts of Parenting a Child with a Disability." *American Journal of Mental Retardation*, 106, 265–286, 2001.

"Semantic Pragmatic Communication Disorder." pediatricneurology.com.

Semantic Pragmatic Disorder Support. "What is Semantic Pragmatic Disorder?" spdsupport.org.uk.

———. "Language Learning Ideas." spdsupport.org.uk.

"Semantic Pragmatic Disorder: What is it?" helpforkidspeech.org.

Sensory Integration International. The Ayres Clinic. "Answers to Frequently Asked Questions." sensoryint.com.

Shackelford, Jo. "State and Jurisdictional Eligibility Definitions for Infants and Toddlers with Disabilities Under IDEA." National Early Childhood Technical Assistance Center. *NECTAC Notes*, no. 21, July 2006.

Sharp, Margo. "Semantic Pragmatic Disorder." American Hyperlexia Association. hyperlexia.org.

Shellenbarger, Sue. "Companies are Offering Assistance to Parents of Kids with Disabilities." *Wall Street Journal Online*. October 14, 2005. careerjournal.com.

———. "New Rulings Clarify Job Protections for Parents of Children with Disabilities." *Wall Street Journal*. July 6, 2006.

Shih, Chilin, and Greg Kochanski. "Prosody and Prosodic Models." Prosody tutorial at 7th International Conference on Spoken Language Processing. Denver, September 16, 2002.

Siegel, Lawrence M. *The Complete IEP Guide: How to Advocate for Your Special Ed Child*. Berkeley, CA: Nolo, 2005.

SIL International. "What Is a Phoneme?" sil.org.

Simms, Mark. Interview. February 15, 2006.

Simpson, Joy, and Mabel L. Rice. "Top Ten Things You Should Know About Children with Specific Language Impairment." Merrill Advanced Studies Center. The University of Kansas. merrill.ku.edu.

Smith, Patricia McGill. "You Are Not Alone: For Parents When They Learn That Their Child Has a Disability." News Digest 20, Third Edition, 2003. National Dissemination Center for Children with Disabilities.

Snowling, Margaret J., and Marianna E. Hayiou-Thomas. "The Dyslexia Spectrum: Continuities Between Reading, Speech and Language Impairments." *Topics in Language Disorders*, vol. 26 (2), 110–126, April/June 2006.

SpeechEasy. "SpeechEasy Fluency Devices." speecheasy.com.

Speechville Express. "Insurance." speechville.com.

———. "Reasons for Insurance Denials." speechville.com.

Spolter, Loring, N. "Employment Law Protections for Parents of Disabled and Ill Children." wrightslaw.com.

Spracher, Mary M. "Learning About Literacy: SLPs Play Key Role in Reading, Writing." *ASHA Leader Online.* asha.org.

Stackhouse, Joy. "Children with Apraxia and Reading, Writing and Spelling Difficulties." apraxia-kids.org.

———. "Phonological Awareness: Connecting Speech and Literacy Problems." *Perspectives in Applied Phonology.* B. Hodson and M. L. Edwards (Eds.). Gaithersburg, MD: Aspen Publications, 1997.

Stoll, Andrew L. *The Omega-3 Connection.* New York: Fireside, 2002.

Stuttering Foundation of America. "Seven Ways to Help the Child Who Stutters." Compiled by Barry Guitar and Edward G. Contuve. stutteringhelp.org.

Styba, Leslie. "Disorder vs. Delay." The Speech-Language Pathology Website. home.ica.net/~frd/anchor7.htm.

Survey of Physicians and Nurses. Kaiser Family Foundation and Harvard University School of Public Health. Menlo Park, CA: Henry J. Kaiser Family Foundation, July 1999. kff.org.

Tansella, C. Z. "Psychological Factors and Chronic Illness in Childhood." *European Psychiatry,* 10, 6, 297–309, 1995.

Taylor, David. "Essential Fatty Acids, Diet and Developmental Disorders." positivehealth.com

Therapeutic Interventions of Georgia. "What Is Sensory Integration?" tiofga.com.

"Therapeutic Listening." Abilities. abilitiesinfo.com.

"Treatment of Cerebral Palsy." originsofcerebralpalsy.com.

Truax, Darci. Interview. July 16, 2006.

Twenty-Fourth Annual Report to Congress on the Implementation of the Individuals with Disabilities Education Act, 2002. Executive Summary.

Twenty-Sixth Annual Report to Congress on the Implementation of the Individuals with Disabilities Education Act, 2004, vol. 1.

UCLID Desk Reference on Language and Speech Milestones. uclid.org.

Ummeed Child Development Center. "Occupational Therapy." ummeed.org.

University of Maryland Medical Center. "Omega-6 Fatty Acids." umm.edu.

U.S. Department of Education. Office of Special Education and Rehabilitation Services. "A Guide to the IEP." July 2000.

———. National Center for Education Statistics (2006). *Digest of Education Statistics,* (NCES 2006-030), Table 50, 2005.

U.S. Department of Health and Human Services. "The National Survey on Children with Special Health Care Needs." Health Resources and Services Administration. Maternal and Child Health Bureau, 2001.

U.S. Department of Health and Human Services and U.S. Environmental Protection Agency. "2004 EPA and FDA Advice for Women Who Might Become Pregnant, Women Who Are Pregnant, Nursing Mothers, Young Children." cfsan.fda.gov.

U.S. Government Accountability Office. "Report to the Ranking Minority Member." Committee on Health, Education, Labor, and Pensions, U.S. Senate. Individuals with Disabilities Education Act. December 2005.

U.S. Office of Personnel Management. "What Is a Health Care Flexible Spending Account?" Federal Flexible Spending Account Program. fsafeds.com.

University of Maryland Hearing and Speech Sciences. "What Can I Expect When I Come for a Hearing Test?" bsos.umd.edu.

University of Nebraska-Lincoln. Hattie B. Munroe Barkley Memorial Augmentative and Alternative Communication Centers. "Activities to Encourage Communication."

Upledger, John E. "Research and Observations That Support The Existence of a Craniosacral System." upledger.com.

Upledger Institute. "Meet the Staff: John E. Upledger." upledger.com

Veale, Tina K. "Targeting Temporal Processing Deficits Through FastForword: Language Therapy with a New Twist." *Language, Speech and Hearing Services in Schools*, vol. 30, no. 4, 353–62, October 1999.

"Velopharyngeal Insufficiency." healthatoz.com.

Vignola, Denise. "Strategies and Suggestions for Dealing with Semantic Pragmatic Disorder." Semantic Pragmatic Disorder Web Page. geocities .com/denisev2.

Voress, Judith K., and Nils A. Pearson. *Early Childhood Development Chart*. Austin, TX: Pro-Ed, 2003.

Wajda, Veronica, and Kent Brorson. "Referrals for Speech and Language Services: Are Medical Students/Residents Prepared?" Presented at the American Speech-Language-Hearing Association convention, New Orleans, 2001.

Washington University, School of Medicine. "Pediatric Spinal Cord Rehabilitation." neuro.wustl.edu.

Waterman, Betsy B. "Assessing Children for the Presence of a Disability." National Information Center for Children and Youth with Disabilities. nichcy.org.

Webster, Richard I., and Michael I. Shevell. "Neurobiology of Specific Language Impairment." *Journal of Child Neurology*, 19(7): 471–481, 2004.

Wellman-Bush, Robyn. "Activities/Games/Ideas for Articulation Therapy." angelfire.com/nm2/speechtherapyideas.

Whitely, Paul, Jacqui Rodgers, Dawn Savery, and Paul Shattock. "A Gluten-Free Diet As an Intervention for Autism and Associated Spectrum Disorders: Preliminary Findings." *Autism*, vol. 3, no. 1, 45–65, 1999.

Williams, Michael B. "AAC 101: A Crash Course for Beginners." Augmentative Communication Inc. augcominc.com.

Willinger, Ulrike, Esther Brunner, Gabriele Diendorfer-Kadner, et al. "Behavior in Children with Language Development Disorders." *The Canadian Journal of Psychiatry*, October 2003.

Wright, Peter. Interview. September 12, 2006.

Zero To Three. "Learning to Talk." zerotothree.org.

Zimcosky, Leslie. Interview. July 9, 2006.

Index